GOOD MANUFACTURING PRACTICE IN TRANSFUSION MEDICINE

DEVELOPMENTS IN HEMATOLOGY AND IMMUNOLOGY

Volume 29

The titles published in this series are listed at the end of this volume.

Good Manufacturing Practice in Transfusion Medicine

Proceedings of the Eighteenth International Symposium on Blood Transfusion, Groningen 1993, organized by the Red Cross Blood Bank Groningen-Drenthe

edited by

C. Th. SMIT SIBINGA and P. C. DAS
Red Cross Blood Bank Groningen-Drenthe, The Netherlands

and

H. J. HEINIGER
Swiss Red Cross, Bern, Switzerland

KLUWER ACADEMIC PUBLISHERS
DORDRECHT / BOSTON / LONDON

A C.I.P. Catalogue record for this book is available from the Library of Congress

ISBN 0-7923-3009-9

Published by Kluwer Academic Publishers,
P.O. Box 17, 3300 AA Dordrecht, The Netherlands.

Kluwer Academic Publishers incorporates
the publishing programmes of
D. Reidel, Martinus Nijhoff, Dr W. Junk and MTP Press.

Sold and distributed in the U.S.A. and Canada
by Kluwer Academic Publishers,
101 Philip Drive, Norwell, MA 02061, U.S.A.

In all other countries, sold and distributed
by Kluwer Academic Publishers Group,
P.O. Box 322, 3300 AH Dordrecht, The Netherlands.

Printed on acid-free paper

Baxter

Acknowledgement

This publication has been made possible through the support of Baxter, which is gratefully acknowledged.

CONTENTS

IV. Good Clinical Practice (CGP)

MODERATORS AND SPEAKERS

Moderators

H.J. Heiniger (chairman)	– Swiss Red Cross, Bern, CH
P.C. Das	– Red Cross Blood Bank Groningen-Drenthe, Groningen, NL
H.I. Hannema	– Pharmaceutical Inspection, Amsterdam, NL
P.A. Hoppe	– F.D.A., Rockville, MD, USA
C.Th. Smit Sibinga	– Red Cross Blood Bank Groningen-Drenthe, Groningen, NL
H.J.C. de Wit	– Red Cross Blood Bank Friesland, Leeuwarden, NL
T.F. Zuck	– Hoxworth Blood Center, Cincinnati, OH, USA

Speakers

A.M. Ali	– Canadian Red Cross Society, Hamilton, Ontario, C
S. Arnoldussen	– Pharmaceutical Consultancy Services, Ouderkerk a/d IJssel, NL
T. Caglioti	– Ortho Diagnostic Systems, Raritan, NJ, USA
B. Cuthbertson	– Protein Fractionation Centre, Edinburgh, UK
Y. Dumas	– Baxter SA, Maurepas, F
B. Flan	– Regional Blood Transfusion Centre, Lille, F
L.W. Gormley	– University of Groningen, Faculty of Law, Groningen, NL
N.S. Klazinga	– C.B.O., Utrecht, NL
D.B.L. McClelland	– Edinburgh & S.E. Scotland Blood Transfusion Service, Edinburgh, UK
D.E. Nevalainen	– Abbott Quality Institute, Chicago, IL, USA
J.L. Robins	– New York Blood Center, New York, NY, USA

K. Sazama – University of California Davis Medical Center, Sacramento, CA, USA

B.T. Teague – Gulf Coast Regional Blood Center, Houston, TX, USA

F. Wells – Association of the British Pharmaceutical Industry, London, UK

J.Th.M. de Wolf – University Hospital Groningen, Groningen, NL

Prepared discussants

B.A. Kerner – Octa Pharma, Vienna, A

H. Oehlmann – ICS International AG, Neu-Anspach, D

INTRODUCTION

TQM AND TAYLORISM; HOW THEY COMPARE

H. Bremer

Preface

The industrial world today is divided between two camps: a culture based on the principles of Total Quality Management (TQM), developed in the Far East, and one still strongly influenced by the origins of "Scientific Management", introduced in the West by F.W. Taylor and others at the turn of the century. This divergence will be shown to have arisen in the last forty years, long enough for a new generation of managers and corresponding culture to emerge. The two cultures are so deeply entrenched that it is difficult for one to change to the other. However, there is strong evidence to support the contention that people-oriented TQM is superior, and those companies clinging to Taylor models now face difficult decisions. Actions by Taylor-companies to move to TQM might well be hindered rather than helped by applying present Quality Assurance Standards, developed by Taylor-oriented national and international Standards Institutions.

The world from 1900 up to the 1939-45 war

In the early 1990s industrial production was chaotically organized. In the USA, F.W. Taylor was the leading exponent of production planning to solve the problems: factory layouts were changed, various mechanical processes broken down into required sequences, time spent on each process measured, and stock control of material and finished products introduced etc. The industrial capacity of the world rose enormously at greatly enhanced efficiency and Japan took part in this using more or less the same disciplines. Japan, in fact, became well known for its ability to copy the West. Quality, as a concept, was scarcely understood and, in any event, consumers had little choice. Slowly, as competition grew and profitability was squeezed, quality inspection started with examination of finished goods which was hesitantly extended to incoming material and component supplies. During this phase, workforces were ill-educated (even ilitterate in some instances) and training was limited to very basic schemes for a few of the brightest. The rate of technological change was of course slow, so that very long production runs of unchanged products and processes were possible. In this atmosphere, the new production planning "Scientific Management" was designed by a few "thinkers" and given to the "do-ers" who, for the most part, were caught in soul destroying repetitive operations for which ever increasing speed was sought. There was practically no delegation of authority and responsibility, and comments on the products and processes were not expected from the workforce and indeed were not encouraged. Company managements were not prepared to listen to their workforces who were consequently demotivated. Japan was no exception.

The impact of World War II

Compared with previous conflicts, the weaponry was sophisticated, for instance, the number of aircrafts equipped with electronic guidance. Quality was soon perceived to be poor: equipment did not work in the field and time was essential to put things right. The response of the military, especially the USA and UK, was to impose rigid directives on suppliers covering not only specifications of finished products, but also requiring manufacturers to specify the processes and conditions under which they should be made. These processes had to be approved and were then subject to regular audit. These procedures were covered under what was known as the AQAP (Allied Quality Assurance Publications) Standards. A few "thinkers" were again designing the systems without participation of the "do-ers", but this time also from outside the actual production units. Under wartime conditions, governments could impose this regime on suppliers and it met with considerable success. Japan, of course, along with Germany, was cut off from this development and whatever these two countries did to enhance their own war machines, it was not with access to, or cooperation with, the greatest industrial power, the US.

Post war recovery

The West, including Germany, was still "product-out" driven and started rebuilding or retuning its industrial apparatus. For some decades the problem was shortage of capacity to meet pent-up demand. There was competition but it was very much a sellers market, in still protected home markets. No real change to the pre-war industrial models occurred. Germany, whose industry had been most devastated among Western nations, took the opportunity to modernize its plants and became an early exponent of high-tech product strategies (though largely unchanged in management concepts and procedures). This period saw the beginning of the divergence between Japan and the West.

The US took the same lead in rehabilitating Japan, as it had in its massive support to Europe, and Japan was cut off from most other contacts with the West. American quality experts (notably Juran and Deming) were among the advisers sent and their early teachings on a new philosophy fell on much more fertile ground in Japan than at home. Perhaps part of the explanation lies in the past copying of the West, so that when this aid was offered, was it not the obvious thing to do? Further, Japanese industry was in tatters affording a "green field" for innovative thinking.

Late 1950s, the 60s and early 70s-high growth and increasing competition

Quality

Once the immediate post war demand for basics had been fulfilled, buyers could exercise more choice and quality became much more important as a competitive tool in obtaining business. The response of the West was to capitalize on war time experience and extend the tight inspection and Quality Assurance procedures to civil production. Quality departments flourished and reported directly to the chief executive enhancing their role as an "independent police force". Quality assurance, which for the greater part replaced simple inspection, is a system whereby the customer seeks to dispense with extensive incoming inspection by being "assured" by the supplier that the goods meet the required standard. However, a simple "assurance" is insufficient unless it is backed up by the supplier demonstrating that he has, in effect, accepted and implemented procedures as laid down in national or international QA-standards imposed by the customer. Quality Assurance is thus based on a measure of distrust between the supplier and customer and within the supplier organisation. All these moves were and still are accomplished as add-on functions to the basic Taylor models. Such additions were not, in fact, confined to quality matters and all kinds of new departments, such as for automation, organisation and efficiency, environmental, safety at work, etc. also flourished, all with the same ethos of "thinkers" imposing new and or different standards and auditing disciplines on the "doers". Even though improvements were achieved, the increasingly better educated workforces were more and more demotivated being essentially left out of the process. In fact, Quality Assurance, rigidly and unthinkingly applied, will be a powerful demotivating influence – something that still happens today when the prime objective is mere certification. Also, all these steps could be taken without examining amongst others the culture in a company, organisational matters and fundamental marketability of a product: improving the technical quality of something no-one actually wants.

In Japan, quality was being pursued dramatically different. Quality was perceived as "fit for use" and the customer must be entirely satisfied with a product at an acceptable cost to the supplier. The "use" is determined by the customer and will accommodate luxury and fashion as well as basic needs. This concept is not confined to the relationship between supplier and external customer, but is also applied to internal relationships within the supplier. Each process in the chain is in a supplier/customer mode – which extends to both horizontal and vertical senses within the organisation – and the most important feature is that products in the widest sense are passed from one to the other with the same meaning of "fit for use". Everyone understands and accepts these concepts and realizes that they will be the prime factors in judging performance. Note that in the supplier/customer relationships, the processes are carried on by units enjoying a high degree of autonomy. The process of the unit or department is not rigidly prescribed as in Taylor models, but with a very large input from the unit itself. This requires a much higher level of education and training of the personnel and this fits in very well with the Japanese obsession with education and dissemination of information.

Continuous improvement is also a very fundamental part of the culture. Improvement applies not only to the strictly technical activities, for which mechanical or electrical parameters are well understood, but to all activities at all levels. To arrive at improvement one must first determine priorities derived from "Policy Deployment" and then arrive at something measurable. The personnel themselves devise what the latter should be, for instance a reduction in the number of complaints in a canteen or cleaning service. As soon as a seemingly unimproveable situation has been arrived at, the process itself is looked at afresh. Taylor companies have copied this idea to some extent but the degree of motivation is not so high in heavily prescribed processes and there is some apprehension in drawing attention to shortcomings. The TQM ethos is to encourage exposure of problems as an opportunity for improvement. Matsushita points out that improvement is regarded as a defence of the company and, ipso facto, of the employees. Another way of looking at this is to say that TQM removes a lot of fear and apprehension amongst employees and will thus considerably help in gaining their cooperation.

A spin-off of the TQM approach appears in increased flexibility. The processes, in which the personnel will have made a design contribution leading to good acceptance and understanding, often include some anticipation of changes or substitution of one employee for another (multi function) in cases of absence. When major changes are needed, new products or processes for instance, the personnel feel less apprehensive when process design will again be amendable to a contribution from themselves.

Strategic planning

Strategy has always been the single most important element of any business for as far back as one cares to go, even if it only existed in the mind of the owner. It is therefore pertinent to look at how strategy formulation fits in with TQM, especially as a decision on whether to introduce TQM is essentially strategic. With increasing complexities of the 20th century, particularly in large, divisionalized companies and institutions, "strategic planning" as a special technique began at around the 1960s in the US. General Electric and the consultants McKinsey and Boston Consulting were among the pioneers. However, this work was carried on in comparatively high growth, stable conditions and the microprocessor revolution had not yet arrived. Japan was perceived as a threat but markets were not yet globalized to such a great extent as today. In these circumstances it was not too difficult, through a rigorous examination of markets and internal strengths and weaknesses, to shift emphasis to something more profitable. As all important competitors were operating in a Taylor mode it was not necessary to endure the trauma of major changes in culture, even if anyone had suggested it. Seeing these moves and early successes, many large companies rushed to adopt "strategic planning" but in the classic Taylor way, the addition of new departments, filled with MBAs and PhDs, as "super thinkers". In Japan, the most striking adoption of strategic planning, with or without the US techniques, was in the formulation of plans for massive international expansion. As is now well known, various industries were selected as targets and considerable help was given by the Ministry of Trade and Industry (MITI). That there was a cosy carve-up by "Japan Inc." in which all companies were orchestrated by MITI is, however, a commonly held false belief. In the two prime industry segments targeted – consumer electronics and automobiles – there was intense competition. Matsushita, Sony, Hitachi and Mitsubishi were major players in the former and Toyota, Nissan and Honda in the latter. One of the notable examples of the competition that was to develop later (in the 1980s) was that between Matsushita with VHS and Sony with Betamax for the home video market. Incidentally, Philips with a technically very good V2000 showed just how ill-equipped a Western company can be in playing in this field.

The 1970s and 1980s-turmoil and the triumph of Japan?

Quality

The West perceived that quality was becoming a problem. Japanese reject rates on components soon became so low as to be negligible, while with finished products shed a once popular image of poor copies of the West to become trend setters in the customer's eye. Some Western companies decided to adopt TQM. Introduction was costly but, once fully implemented, results could be seen in improved performance. Such early successful introduction was, however, the exception rather than the rule. Some only saw TQM as the latest vogue and attempted to introduce it in traditional Taylor fashion by hiring a few experts, starting up an improvement program and making a few cosmetic changes, especially those that could be seen externally by the customer. There was no real understanding of the profound cultural and organisational change required internally, nor the need for true involvement of all personnel. For the most part, however, TQM was ignored and the response of many companies in the West was first to retreat from the low end of markets and concentrate efforts on improving the quality of more expensive products. The second move was to enhance the quality "policing" directives still stemming from the wartime experience. Quality Assurance standards were developed, external quality institutions grew in stature and Quality Assurance (QA) certification was eagerly sought. Note, however, that certification may have imprecise meanings. The same level of approval can be spread over different industry segments with varying perceptions of quality. Part of the difficulty may lie in the varying segments with varying perceptions of quality. Part of the difficulty may lie in the varying degree of expertise among the personnel involved in granting certification (registration). None of these measures really solved the competition problem and they did not provide the motivation for self-improvement and continuous improvement. Nevertheless, quality did rise and a company with really poor quality would have been especially improved by fulfilling the certification requirements. Unfortunately, such improvement did not address a variety of demotivating factors affecting the workforce, especially those leading to absenteeism and high turn over of people. Nor did they address the organisation outside the immediate technical sectors and they completely ignored the basic marketability of the products. Moreover, the idea of continuous improvement was made somewhat difficult as some changes that might be necessary for such improvement might run contrary to certification rules. Essentially, the Taylor culture, and also of the related Quality Assurance standards, is not a "listening" one in which all employees are able and perceived to be able to make contributions for the improvement of the products and the processes by which they are made. Japan continued to refine its people and market oriented approach, particularly by extending the idea of quality and improvement to all parts of the organisation. The ability to contribute to improvement is enhanced by the extensive training given to all employees at various stages in their service with the company. For instance, a design engineer may well serve appreciable time in on-the-floor production jobs before turning to design so that unnecessarily difficult assembly tasks can be avoided by attention at the design stage. He may then spend time in other departments (his future internal customers) with similar benefits to the company. Such training is part of the structures that have been evolved to make clear the inter-dependence of the units in a company and how the links between them must be treated in a customer/supplier relationship. Further a link was made between strategy and derived policy to all parts of the organisation. Once overall policy had been established that needed to satisfy the prime product/market objectives, this was translated into policies relevant at successively lower levels (policy deployment) so that each constituent part could make the maximum contribution to success. This overall approach is in fact Total Quality Management TQM. How the two cultures compare in more detail is summed up in Table 1.

Strategic planning

By the late 70s, the heavy investment in personnel for planning made in the West was expected to bear fruit. But by now the environment had changed drastically following the microprocessor based technology explosion and the rapid globalization of markets. Furthermore, the separation of planning and other functions from management did not offer good prospects for success. The literature, and planners themselves, made it abundantly clear that strategy could only be decided by top management; planners could only advise and assist with information and techniques. Nevertheless, many boards of companies with large planning units took no active part in the process and waited for elegant presentations by the planners which they then sometimes scarcely understood. Occasionally and sometimes even frequently, the message of the planners was bleak when there was then a tendency to "shoot the messenger".

The outcome of all this was that many companies were confronted with great difficulties brought about by the rapid environmental changes and very often the appearance of a Japanese company as the main competitor. There was a feeling that strategic planning had failed to deliver and in fairness to managements the planners were having to re-think the techniques that had been more appropriate to stable times. Formal strategic planning in the West thus ended the 80s with an uncertain image of the techniques that had been introduced. However, many could argue that this was brought about more by a failure through incorrect implementation rather than a fault in principle. There is a lesson to be learnt here concerning the introduction of TQM.

The Japanese were, of course, buoyed up by their strategic successes in capturing so many Western markets. They applied the same rigour in quality of strategic planning as in quality of operations and whereas the "what" strategies could have been conceived independent of TQM no doubt the "how" strategies were heavily dependent on it. Nevertheless, the speed of change must have surprised even the Japanese, even though they were prime movers in it, but planning was much more a clear management function so that the same unease could not so easily develop.

The state of the parties for the 1990s

If anything, the turmoil of the 1980s has become worse. The change in East-West relationships has thrown up nationalism with as yet unforeseeable consequences. Also, while no major isolationist practices have, at the time of writing, been put in place, the rumbling noises between the EEC and the US are not comforting. In this difficult scenario, the two cultures – TQM and those companies following Western Taylorism – compete for trade. In this context, the two cultures invariably face each other in global trade whereas non-TQM companies operating locally, and only meeting local competitors, may not yet feel the consequences. However, it can only be a question of time before the latter situation changes. Recently, US president Clinton in his speech at Washington University (Febr. 1993) graphically drew attention to the shrinking globe and the need to compete on an international scale: three quarters of US products are subject to foreign competition. To reach the customer, a "minefield" of competitors must first be crossed. In satisfying the customer, long term continuity will also depend on satisfying or reconciling, a number of other "stake-holders" or agencies linked to the marketplace. Some of these will be supportive, some regulatory, some possibly hostile and others watchful with uncertain intentions. The speed of technological change and political turmoil embrace all.

The crucial point

We have now indeed reached a crucial point. One of the major strategic decisions for Taylor managements, certainly the major decision for them collectively, is how to meet the challenges of the TQM culture. The difficulties experienced in the 80s may have some beneficial effects: managements will take a more active role in planning and some of the old style macho managements have been replaced with better trained people of a different character who will be able to use the analyses made available to them more effectively. For some managements a kind of "post-certification syndrome" has set in: Quality Assurance certificates have been obtained after considerable effort and expense without any tangible improvement in results. What to do next must be the cause of considerable deliberation.

Any company deciding unilaterally to change to a people-oriented TQM style organisation would face considerable problems and uncertainties. The first hurdle is to secure top management *understanding and conviction.* Still today there are a large number of managements who have certainly heard of TQM but who really do not understand it. Just as strategic planning was embraced as something fashionable and must be seen to be being done, TQM is observed but considered as something that can be added to the existing structure. This probably accounts for a large proportion of the reported lack of success with the introduction of TQM – or rather what such managements *think* is TQM. Let us, nevertheless, assume that top managements have correctly taken on board the concept, there will then still be many difficulties:

- Conviction would be needed also of middle and lower management, as well as the shop floor, where deeply entrenched cultures exist and TQM might be seen as a threat. There may be no alternative to replacing some 20–30% of higher and middle management.
- Would the right skills exist for implementation? How long would any action take and at what cost?
- How much current business is dependent on certification by outside standards institutions? Would certification be lost by changes in practice?
- How would customers and suppliers react anyway?

A satisfactory implementation might well take five or ten years rather than months during which time the normal product/market strategies would have to be executed and unexpected problems dealt with. It is a rather daunting task. The size of the task might well prompt a search for less traumatic solutions. The author does not pretend to prescribe what these could be, but the first part of a solution is to recognize the problem, and especially understand what people-oriented TQM really is, and that is a major objective of this paper. Perhaps some imaginative managements will find quicker solutions but, for many, unilateral action will be hindered by external factors. This leads to the question of possible help via Standards Institutions, but this idea is put forward with a certain amount of caution, however, suitable standards could be used as a check-list to help managements to find a solution on how to start. Establishment of TQM through prescriptive directives would be a contradiction in terms of the first order, so that, if Standards Institutions can play a part, it will have to involve considerable innovative thinking as well. We might have to find compromises whereby present certification is acquired along the path to people-oriented TQM. Certification then becomes a milestone and not an end point.

So far, new thinking from Standards Institutions has not been very great. Let the discussions start!

I. Principles of Good Manufacturing Practice (GMP)

STATE OF THE ART AND FUTURE DIRECTIONS A BRIEF OVERVIEW

H.J. Heiniger

Introduction

Good Manufacturing Practice (GMP) and the need for product improvement became a major issue in blood transfusion in many western countries in the late 60s. This was most evident in the United States where a centralized agency, the Food and Drug Administration (FDA), was empowered to control not only the manufacturers of drugs but also blood banks and the manufacturers of products originating from human blood and its components. Today, most countries have created such agencies which control (more or less intensively) the activities of blood banks and fractionation facilities. This appears to be related to several factors:

1. An ever increasing number of safety tests that have to be performed, implying that the possibility of errors also increases.
2. The increasing complexity of technology and equipment
3. A shortage of appropriately trained laboratory personnel in some countries.
4. The development of new products for diseases for which no, or only limited, treatments exist.

To satisfy the ever increasing demand for safety and quality, well-planned and carefully managed Quality Assurance (QA) programs have to be implemented, not only to guarantee safety and quality, but also to prevent, detect and correct errors, with the goal of prevention, rather than retrospective detection.

The public (i.e. the patients) has the legitimate right to demand that the risks associated with blood transfusion are kept as low as possible. These risks are not insignificant, as demonstrated in the case of red cell transfusion. It has been documented that minor transfusion reactions (fever, chills, urticaria) may occur as frequently as 1/100 units transfused, hemolytic transfusion reactions in 1/6,000 units, fatal hemolytic reactions in 1/100,000 units, hepatitis C transmission in 1/10,000 units, hepatitis B in less than 1/200,000 units. HIV varies very much from region to region, but the US average for example has been estimated to be approximately 1/250,000 units transfused.

In this symposium experts in GMP, Good Clinical Practice (GCP) and QA will describe in detail the various aspects of QA programs and activities; I therefore will limit myself to a few remarks.

Quality Assurance program

Potential public health consequences require that all establishments which are engaged in any aspect of blood transfusion implement and invest in QA regardless of their size. This, as other speakers will demonstrate, requires an enormous commitment of time, personnel and financial resources. It particularly requires a specialized QA unit, often also called Quality Control unit, although the latter term refers more to technical aspects. QA indeed encompasses all activities and all persons of any given establishment.

The following paragraphs, will give a brief outline of the various components and activities of a comprehensive QA program as presently visualized by various government agencies and international organizations involved in blood transfusion.

Reporting responsibilities

The QA unit should report to the top management, i.e., to the responsible head, the individual who holds the establishment license and represents a firm in all its regulatory activities. It is important that the QA unit reports to management independently from production and ensures that production follows GMP accurately. If necessary, the QA unit must have the authority to stop production or release of a product, without considering economic aspects.

Standard Operating Procedures (SOPs)

The QA unit is responsible for ensuring that SOPs exist for all manufacturing procedures including, but not limited to, collection, testing, processing, product release, record keeping, etc. The actual contents of the SOPs may be formulated by the appropriate production and operational units, but the QA unit formally approves each single SOP, thus ensuring that its intended purposes and processes are properly validated. In addition, the QA unit identifies the responsible person for each procedure and certifies that the persons are adequately trained and supervised. This is accomplished through proficiency and competency testing. All SOPs should be on file with the QA department or unit in the form of a master copy. In this symposium, the details of these functions and activities of the QA unit will be described further.

Training and education

The QA unit plays a central role in the formulation and approval of the training and educational programs of an establishment. Such programs should include, but are not restricted to: orientation of new employees; GMP training; SOP training (formulation and implementation); technical and operational training; training of supervisors and managers; QA training; and, computer record keeping training.

It is well known that in many cases of process breakdown and errors, insufficient training of personnel can be identified as the main cause of the problem. Therefore, the audit of training is a critical function of the QA unit, and it must ensure that all employees undergo continuous training.

Competency evaluation and proficiency testing.

Competency evaluation and proficiency tests must be conducted under the supervision of the QA unit if one is to have a truly comprehensive training program. Adequate files should be maintained on results of the competency tests, since they provide the necessary documentation to correct individual or group performance problems, hopefully before actual errors in the production process occur.

Proficiency testing procedures must ensure that the samples are tested by *all* personnel performing routine tests and using routine testing equipment. In case of unsuccessful proficiency test performance, the QA unit must have systematic written plans for remedial action.

Validation

The definition of this activity dates back only a few years. But today many countries in Europe, like the USA, have issued clear-cut guidelines regarding proper validation procedures for any given process or system. It is one of the most important activities of the QA unit to ensure that adequate and generally accepted validation procedures have been performed and have been sanctioned by the regulatory authorities.

Validation requirements will undoubtedly be tightened further in the future since serious problems in blood transfusion in the past were often caused by absent or inappropriate validation procedures.

Equipment

An essential component of the QA program is the validation, maintenance and monitoring of all equipment within an establishment. For each piece of equipment written procedures (SOPs) have to be available, and a reporting system regarding malfunctioning or out-of calibration status has to be established by the QA unit. Computer systems which are used in manufacturing or for testing purposes are also subject to rigid validation procedures. For example, the American regulatory agency FDA has issued specific requirements for computer systems used in blood collecting and processing activities.

Complaints and adverse reactions

The QA programs must provide assurance that all complaints and accident reports from the users of the blood products are received promptly by the manufacturer. Since some adverse reactions may be life-threatening, disabling or even fatal, procedures have to be in place to document such incidents in a timely manner and to trigger immediate corrective actions, including interruption of production, product recalls and/or withdrawal from the market.

The feedback of all information regarding complaints, reports of accidents, errors and adverse reactions to QA represents an essential element of a QA program, since without thorough investigation of these incidents the cause of the problems remains unidentified and thus cannot be corrected. Such corrective actions may involve personnel retraining, changes in the manufacturing processes or even substantial system redesigns.

Record keeping and management

A properly validated record keeping system has to be approved by the QA unit in accordance with international guidelines, covering all steps from the donor interview to the distribution of the final manufactured product. It is particularly important that electronic or computerized record keeping systems be properly validated, although such a process requires an enormous technical and logistical effort.

Most regulatory agencies have issued specific requirements regarding the time for which records have to be kept on file (in most cases 10 years). In the past, insufficient compliance with required record keeping has led to temporary or permanent closure of blood banks.

Product release procedures

A "lot" of product is represented by all the components (e.g. red cell concentrate, platelets, plasma, etc.) prepared from a simple unit of whole blood with a unique lot number, usually assigned to at the moment of collection. The QA unit must implement procedures ensuring that the lot number assignments are accurate during each step of testing and processing so as to be assured that any discrepancies or failures of a lot, or unit are immediately detected and that corrective action is taken, including the autoclaving and discarding of units unsuitable for transfusion.

Strict labelling procedures are crucial to warrant the safety and quality of any product issued by a blood processing facility, including the collection center per se; therefore, the QA unit has to design written protocols to ensure that procedures in labelling, packaging and shipping are meticulously followed in order to minimize the risks of errors.

Since blood components are often converted from one product to another, the QA unit has to take all necessary measures to assure that relabelling procedures are subject to the same control mechanisms and record keeping procedures as the initial labelling of the blood and its components. Prior to release, all steps leading up to labelling should be reviewed and verified independently in order to exclude any errors.

As an example, it is common knowledge that the cause of fatal hemolytic reactions in many cases is due to errors related to labelling, which can be avoided through a comprehensive QA program.

Quality assurance audits

As a logical consequence of all the responsibilities and requirements that a QA program has to assume and fulfil, appropriate QA audits, internal and external, should be conducted periodically to evaluate the effectiveness of the QA system within an establishment. Some regulatory agencies and international organizations have already issued guidelines which describe in detail such audits, which are specifically addressed in this Symposium. One important requirement of a QA audit is that although the auditors have to be very knowledgable regarding the specific processes under review, they should not be responsible for performing the procedures which they audit. This requirement is often not easily fulfilled, due to limitations in human resources.

The results of such audits including a plan for possible corrective actions, should be made available not only to the head of the QA unit, but also to the top management for review.

QA audits should be structured in a way so as to identify the critical control points in every single operation of a blood processing establishment, including quality control, donor selection, blood collection practices, component manufacturing, product testing, storage and distribution methods, lot release, and logistics and computer operations. Since audit procedures will vary in their complexity according to the specific details and size of an establishment, it is unavoidable that in each case a customized system has to be developed.

Conclusions and perspective

Even in this brief overview of the components of a QA program, it becomes readily evident that probably only a few blood banks have implemented such programs today.

The formulation of GMP has originated within the blood bank community out of genuine concern for the safety and quality of their products and services. Nowadays, rigorous quality assurance programs are being imposed, involving endless new requirements, by regulatory agencies worldwide. As examples, I may mention the substantial volumes of "Rules Governing Medicinal Products in the European Community", issued in recent years by the EC's Committee for Proprietary Medicinal Products (CPMP). Another and more subtle example is the recent document of the American FDA, which now talks about cGMP, i.e. *current* Good Manufacturing Practices, which implies that GMP, once defined for a process, must undergo constant revisions to adapt to the fulminant, progressive growth of new technologies, tests and products.

These developments, although contributing to much desired improvements in safety and quality, also bring the blood processing establishments to a dilemma:

Since such programs often now called TQM, Total Quality Management programs, are very personnel intensive, they require the highest qualified human recources and are therefore extremely cost intensive. These future cost increases must be recovered through the price structure of the services and products provided. At a time when every government wants to reduce health care costs, it remains unclear how ambitious TQM programs will be funded in the future.

Another example is the recent creation of GCP, Good Clinical Practice (GCP), which will require enormous efforts to develop a consensus for concepts and guidelines acceptable to manufacturers and clinicians alike. This process alone will represent a major task for transfusion medicine.

Acknowledgements

The author wishes to thank Dr. R.G. Westphal for critically reviewing the manuscript. The competent and efficient secretarial assistance of Mrs. D. Moser is gratefully acknowledged.

List of selected references, guidelines and governmental rules

Since the publications listed below pertain to all paragraphs in this Chapter they are not cited in specific places in the text. They are intended to be useful to readers who want to familiarize themselves in depth with the topics of GMP and QA.

a. General references

Bartlett R. Leadership for quality. ASM News 1991;57:15-21.

DeBoy J, Jarboe B. Government-mandated cytology proficiency testing: Practical, equitable and defensible standards. ORB 1991:152-61.

Juran, J. Quality control handbook. McGraw-Hill, New York NY ,1974.

Kritchevsky S,. Simmons B. Continuous quality improvement: Concepts and applications for physician care. JAMA 1991;266:1817-23.

Milakovich ME. Creating a total quality health care environment. Health Care Manage Rev 1991;16(2):9-20.

McLaughlin CP, Kaluzny AD. Total quality management in health: Making it work. Health Care Manage Rev 1990;15(3):7-14.

Rosvoll R (ed). Accreditation requirements manual of the American Association of Blood Banks. American Association of Blood Banks, Arlington VA 1990.

Walker R (ed). Technical manual. American Association of Blood Banks, Arlington VA 1990.

Julius C, Westphal RG. The safety of blood components and derivatives. Hematology/Oncology Clinics of North America 1992;6(5):1057-77.

b. Documents issued by the Council of Europe, Health Division, F-67075 Strasbourg Cedex France

Recommendation No. R(86)6. Guidelines for the preparation, quality control and use of fresh frozen plasma (FFP), 1986.

Recommendation No. R(88)4. Responsibilities of health authorities in the field of blood transfusion, 1988.

Recommendation No. R(90)9 + Report. Plasma products and European self-sufficiency, 1990.

Guide to preparation, use and quality assurance of blood components, 1991.

c. Documents issued by the Commission of the European Community, Rue de la Loi 200, B-1049 Bruxelles, Belgium

The rules governing medicinal products for human use in the European Community. Volume I. Catalogue number CO-71-91-631-EN-C.

Notice to applicants for marketing authorisations for medicinal products for human use in the Member States of the Community. Volume II. Catalogue number CB-55-89-293-EN-C.

Guidelines on the quality, safety and efficacy of medicinal products for human use. Volume III. Catalogue number CB-55-89-843-EN-C.

Addendum (July 1990) CB-59-90-936-EN-C.

Addendum No. 2 (May 1992) CO-75-92-558-EN-C.

Good Manufacturing Practice for medical products. Volume IV. Catalogue number CO-71-91-760-EN-C.

Council directive 89/381/EEC of 14 June 1989, extending the scope of Directives 65/65/EEC and 75/319/EEC on the approximation of provisions laid down by law, regulation or administrative action relating to proprietary medicinal products and laying down special provisions for medicinal products derived from human blood and human plasma (O.J. No. L181 of 28.6.89).

Note for Guidance. Medicinal products derived from human blood and plasma in Volume III of the rules governing medicinal products in the European Community, addendum No. 2. Catalogue number CO-75-92-558-EN-C.

Note for Guidance. Validation of virus removal and inactivation procedures in Volume III of the rules governing medicinal products in the European Community, addendum No. 2. Catalogue number CO-75-92-558-EN-C.

111/3232/92. Manufacture of products derived from human blood or human plasma, Annex to the EC guide to the GMP.

d. Selected Documents issued by the World Health Organization, WHO, 20, Ave Appia, CH-1211 Geneva, Switzerland

Lab/89.5. Minimum targets for blood transfusion services. (Available in English, French, Spanish).

Lab/89.6. Consensus statement on accelerated strategies to reduce the risk of transmission of HIV by blood transfusion. (Available in English, French, Spanish).

Lab/89.7. Essential blood components, plasma derivatives and substitutes. (Available in English, French, Spanish).

Lab/89.8. Essential consumables and equipment of a blood transfusion service. (Available in English, French, Spanish).

Lab/89.9. Use of plasma substitutes and plasma in developing countries. (Available in English, French, Spanish).

Lab/89.10. Guidelines for the appropriate use of blood. (Available in English, French, Spanish).

WHO, 1990. ISBN92-4-154406-6. Management of Blood Transfusion Services.

LBS/91.1. Consensus statement on screening of blood donations for infectious agents transmissible through blood transfusion. (Available in English, French, Spanish).

WHO, 1992. Guidelines for the organization of a blood transfusion service.

WHO/LBS/92.5. Viral inactivation of blood and blood products, by Dr H Suomela, Finland.

WHO/LBS/92.6. Report of the GBSI Informal Consultation on "Assessment of training needs in transfusion medicine".

WHO/LBS/92.7. Report of the GBSI Informal Consultation on "Costing of blood transfusion services".

WHO, 1993. Guidelines for quality assurance programs for blood transfusion services.

Requirements for the collection, processing and quality control of blood, blood components and plasma derivatives. (A revised edition will be published in 1993).

e. Documents issued by the US Health and Human Services, Food and Drug Administration, Center of Biologics Evaluation and Research (HFM-635), 8800 Rockville Pike, Bethesda, BD 20892

Title 21, Code of Federal Regulations, Parts 210, 211, 600, 606, 610, 640, 660.

Center for Drugs and Biologics and Center for Devices and Radiological Health (CDRH), Guideline on general principles of process validation (May 1987).

FDA 91-4179. CDRH, Medical device good manufacturing practices manual, 56th edition (August 1991).

FDA Compliance program guidance manual, blood and blood products, 7342-001 (1992), 7342.002 (1991).

FDA Compliance policy guide, FDA access to results of quality assurance program audits and inspections, 7151.02 (1989).

FDA Memorandum. April 6, 1988, Control of unsuitable blood and blood products.

FDA Memorandum. March 20, 1991, Deficiencies relating to the manufacture of blood and blood components.

Federal Register, Volume 43, No. 190, Friday, September 29, 1978. Human and veterinary drugs, current good manufacturing practice in manufacture, processing, packing, or holding, 45013-45087.

Federal Register, Volume 40, No. 223, Tuesday, November 18, 1975. Human blood and blood products, collection, storage and processing, 53532-53544.

Federal Register, Volume 57, No. 40, Friday, February 28, 1992. Clinical laboratory improvement amendments of 1988, Final Rule, 7002-7288.

DEFINITIONS IN QUALITY ASSURANCE AND QUALITY MANAGEMENT

C.Th. Smit Sibinga, W.P.A. van der Tuuk Adriani

Introduction

Like in many other fields there is in the concept of Quality Assurance (QA) much confusion because of a lack of understanding and an inappropriate communication due to absence of definitions of key-terminology. Where QA in transfusion medicine is concerned with every aspect of transfusion practice and applies to all activities of a blood transfusion service or blood bank, from identification of potential donors, collection of blood and preparation of blood products to ensuring the best, safest and most appropriate use of blood and blood products in the clinic [1], there are many key-issues and terminologies involved which deserve a clear and unequivocal definition.

The conceptual starting point is a Quality System (QS) based on Organization Wide Quality Assurance (OWQA) or Total Quality Management (TQM). OWQA/TQM reflects the institute's or organization's quality policy dealing with personnel, facilities, equipment, safety, product design, purchasing, good manufacturing/laboratory and clinical practice, quality control, quality assurance, storage, distribution, optimal use, consultative services, administration and all related functions.

Such a QA should be based on well defined and accepted standards [2]:
- Standards for procedures and processes;
- Standards for quality control;
- Standards for services.

Examples of such standards are:
- NEN-ISO 9000 series;
- Current Good Manufacturing Practice guidelines;
- Current Good Laboratory Practice guidelines;
- Current Good Hospital/Clinical Practice guidelines;
- Standards for Blood Banks (AABB, USA);
- Normen voor Bloedbanken (NVB/Federatie, NL).

The main elements of an OWQA/TQM based QS are:
- Personnel, trained and motivated;
- Standards;

- Documentation;
- Quality control;
- Quality monitoring;
- Quality assurance;
- Error policy;
- Evaluation and audit.

They key element, however, is dedicated, motivated and professional leadership. Whatever is instituted, implemented and evaluated, personnel will determine whether a quality system or QA program will be effective and successful. Attitude and mentality are of paramount importance, where errors will occur and therefore need attention for prevention leading to improvement in quality. If we accept that errors in the field of transfusion medicine are the primary cause of morbidity and mortality and implicitly reflect a deviation from a standard procedure, then the necessary elements of a QA program are readily apparent and will provide means for error control (prevention and an efficient quality management system.

Focused on the objective of a safe and effective transfusion practice, these necessary elements are:

- Standards and Standard Operating Procedures (SOPs);
- Job descriptions;
- Teaching and training;
- Control of equipment (Equipment Operating Procedures (EOPs)) and reagents;
- Monitoring and evaluation of performance of personnel, equipment and reagents;
- Monitoring and evaluation of efficacy (including safety) of end products.

Definitions

When written up, agreed upon and accepted in consensus, definitions will provide a workable basis for mutual understanding, communication, evaluation and exchange of information and expertise.

Quality: The consistent and reliable performance of services or products in conformity with specified standards.

Quality assurance: The creation and operation of standards, programs and effective management systems to ensure quality, to be achieved by application of Good Manufacturing/Laboratory/Clinical Practice (GMP/GLP/GCP).

Standards: Criteria against which processes, products and services can be measured qualitatively and/or quantitatively.

Policy: This comprises the stated aims, objectives or standards adopted by an institution or organization. These may be determined institutionally, locally or regionally, professionally, nationally or internationally.

Good Manufacturing Practice: All elements in establishing practice which will collectively lead to final products or services consistently meeting expected specifications.

Quality control: That part of a quality assurance program which consists of (retrospective) tests or measures which must be completed with satisfactory results before proceeding further in a given process, and which demonstrates compliance with certain defined limits and specifications.

Quality monitoring: That part of a quality assurance program concerned with maintenance and improvement of quality which deals with the identification and use of indicators to detect variations from standards or specifications.

Guidelines: Recommendations as part of a quality assurance program which are not binding nor compulsory, but embody optimal approaches and considerations.

Validation: That part of a quality assurance program which evaluates in advance the steps involved in operational procedures or product preparation to ensure quality, effectiveness and reliability.

Proficiency testing: An external assessment of the ability of staff to undertake a series of prescribed tests.

Internal quality control: Routine in-process check points defined by Standard Operating Procedures (SOPs) that confirm the validity of the procedure every time it is carried out.

Audit/Inspection: A formal and objective review according to the adopted standards within the quality assurance program to identify problems and approaches to their resolutions.
Audits/inspections can be internal (self-inspection) or external (peer-inspection).

Error: An inadvertent or unauthorized deviation from a standard procedure.

Accreditation: Formal acknowledgement of compliance with accepted standards for procedures, activities or services upon audit or inspection by an authorized institute or organization.

Certificate: Document signed and dated on behalf of an authorized institute or organization to confirm accreditation.

Some fundamental statements

Although the definitions in principle do provide a workable basis for mutual understanding, communication, evaluation and exchange of information and expertise within the framework of OWQA/TQM, it seems appropriate to quote some fundamental statements. These provide a perspective of relevance to any quality assurance program:

- People are the most valuable and important resource.
- Achievements, maintenance and improvement of quality demand that staff at all levels show commitment to the common goal of quality.
- All personnel should be conscious of the implications of the work they are involved in, and aware of the importance of applied quality assurance.

- It is the responsibility of management to ensure that all human resources are used in the most efficient, cost-effective and ethical manner.
- Failure to maintain and improve quality is usually the result of human error, carelessness, or lack of understanding, rather than technological problems.
- It is essential that the application of quality assurance principles (quality management) has a demonstrable impact on an institution's operations and practices.
- Collection and documentation of information, as an integral part of quality management, must be purposeful and relevant to policy. Its influence on procedures must be apparent to the staff involved.
- Ultimate responsibility for implementing, maintaining and improving quality assurance procedures rests with a designated quality assurance officer, who should be accountable directly to the director.
- Sound management practice dictates that any remedial action be implemented only after discussion with the head of the department concerned.
- Unless the fundamental importance of TQM is fully appreciated, the costs of its application may be a cause of concern.

References

1. Guidelines for quality assurance programs for blood transfusion services. World Health Organization, Geneva 1993.
2. Smit Sibinga CTh, Das PC. Standards, inspection and accreditation mechanisms in transfusion medicine. In: Smit Sibinga CTh, Das PC, Cash JD (eds). Transfusion medicine: Fact and fiction. Kluwer Academic Publ. Dordrecht/Boston/London 1992: 71-6.

THE QUALITY ASSURANCE CONCEPT

J.L. Robins

Introduction

The concept of Quality Assurance (QA) for blood establishments has been evolving since 1990.

In anticipation of the regulators (FDA) issuing guidelines, industry initiated two separate programs. The Council of Community Blood Centers (CCBC) developed a current Good Manufacturing Practice (cGMP) course for all blood establishments. American Association of Blood Banks (AABB) established the Technical Quality Assurance Committee to develop a self-assessment manual and QA manual for all blood establishments.

In January, 1992, the FDA conducted an open workshop on QA for blood establishments. A draft guideline document was distributed prior to the workshop for discussion. The draft document was very comprehensive and, as industry had predicted, emphasized cGMPs, self-audit and the importance of a written QA manual.

During the same period, industry and regulators were learning about Total Quality Management (TQM). TQM was defined as a new approach to management, which had as a goal producing high quality products and providing high quality service to meet or exceed customer demands. Management recognized that to achieve the quality it was seeking, an organizationwide commitment to quality was needed.

Both industry and the regulators benefited from their new awareness of TQM. The work products from the industry efforts and the regulators included many of the basic concepts embodied in TQM. For example:

- Work is a process. In order to achieve an agreed upon level of quality in the output of that process, the process must be in control.
- Supplier qualification is an important component of the quality of the final product.
- Error prevention is preferred over error detection.

On June 17, 1993, the Draft *Guideline for quality assurance in blood establishments* was issued by FDA's Center for Biologics Evaluation and Research. These guidelines provided a comprehensive summary of what QA in blood establishments should include. Certainly, QA in blood establishments had moved from concept to reality.

Quality Assurance guidelines

The draft QA guidelines states the following:

"To ensure the continued safety of the nation's blood supply, it is essential that blood establishments implement effective control over manufacturing processes and systems. FDA believes that this can be accomplished by each blood establishment developing a well planned, written and managed QA program designed to recognize and prevent the cause of recurrent deficiencies in blood establishment performance. The goals of QA are to decrease significantly errors, ensure credibility of test results, implement effective manufacturing process and system controls, and ensure continued product safety and quality." [1]

To meet these current standards of excellence necessary for blood establishments, we must implement a QA program that is broader in scope than "traditional quality assurance". We must implement OrganizationWide Quality Assurance (OWQA)/Total Quality Management (TQM). Everyone in the organization must accept responsibility for providing the highest quality products and services.

Using the QA guidelines as reference, the following issues will be addressed:

- Redefining quality assurance
- QA program
- Training for QA

Redefining Quality Assurance

QA must be integrated with other strategic business objectives and include nonfactory/nonlaboratory areas. QA can no longer consist of only inspection and testing, but must be built into the manufacturing process at the earliest point. A total systems approach should be used.

It is critical that "quality consciousness" be developed in every employee. Each employee must understand his/her role in controlling process variation from planned design requirements and helping the organization to attain consistent, predictable levels of quality. Every employee should be involved in continuous improvement. A formalized process improvement activity should be in place to facilitate that continuous improvement.

The redefined QA concept must incorporate current Good Manufacturing Practice (cGMP) requirements, including:

- Organizational issues
- Documentation/Recordkeeping/Record review
- Education/Training/Personnel selection
- Validation/Calibration/PM/Proficiency testing
- Incident/Error/Accident review
- Supplier qualification

- Label control/Process control
- Internal assessment

Also, the redefined QA system should include an element of product assurance which assures customer needs are determined, translated into design requirements and met. Product assurance requires that products are manufactured in a GMP environment.

A critical component of an integrated QA system is the requirement that all feedback from customers and incident review is incorporated into the process improvement cycle. The final critical component of the integrated QA system is a comprehensive written internal audit/assessment program. These audits should evaluate/assess Critical Control Points (CCPs) and Key Elements (KEs) for each of the major systems. This redefined, integrated QA system is called OWQA/TQM. OWQA includes Quality Control (QC), cGMPs and Product Assurance (PA).

Quality control is the minimum type of quality program. Consisting of inspection and testing, QC has limited provision for feedback with design/planning phase. QC does not prevent, it detects.

cGMPs are much broader in scope than QC. cGMPs emphasize all aspects of production. For example, process control, validation, documentation, internal assessment, error/accident capture, etc. Certainly cGMPs include customer feedback, corrective action and process improvement. cGMPs do not emphasize product design.

Product assurance focuses on assuring that a product meets customer requirements, meets company quality claims and is manufactured by a process that is in compliance. See Table 1.

Table 1. **Redefined quality assurance.**

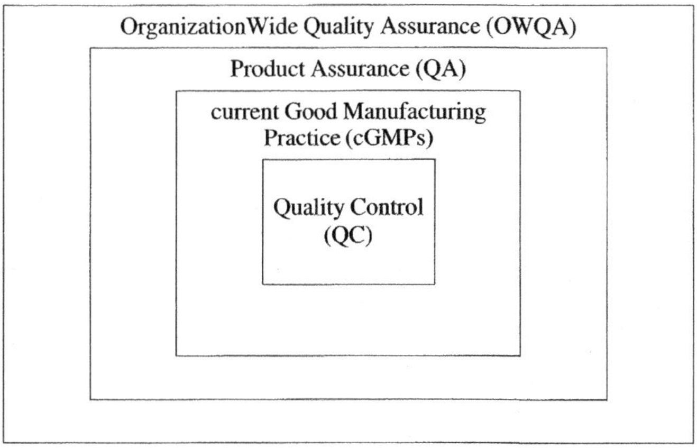

Table 2. **Quality Assurance program overview.**

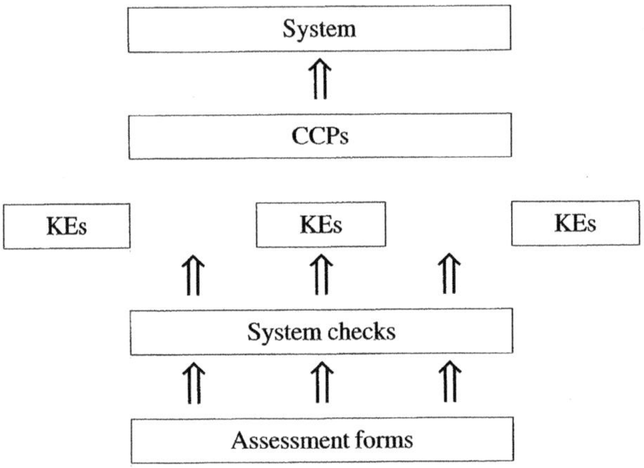

Table 3. **Quality Assurance program (CCPs)**

A. Organizational issues
B. Documentation / Recordkeeping / Record review
C. Education / Training / Personnel selection
D. Validation / Calibration / PM / Proficiency testing
E. Incident / Error / Accident review
F. Process control
G. Supplier qualification
H. Label control
I. Internal assessment
J. Process improvement

Quality Assurance program

The QA guidelines describe the QA program as follows:

"An organization's comprehensive system for manufacturing safe and effective quality products according to regulatory standards including preventing, detecting and correcting deficiencies that may compromise product quality." [1]

Using the QA guidelines and the AABB self-assessment manual as reference documents, blood establishments can define a QA program using the following process:

1. Identify the major systems

Within blood services each major operation is defined as a system. The major systems are quality management, donor suitability, blood collection, component processing, testing, review and labelling, storage and distribution, compatibility testing, blood administration, investigation of adverse reactions and information management. Within each system a number of processes and subprocesses can be described.

2. Identify critical control points (CCPs) , key elements (KEs), system checks

CCPs are major/critical processes within a system, the correct performance of which are necessary to assure the quality of the finished product/service. KEs are steps leading to the CCPs that must be managed to assure error-free processes/subprocesses. System checks are specific activities/tasks to monitor KEs, CCPs and ultimately, system function.

3. Identify assessment forms

These forms are tools to be used in assessing/evaluating the systems. These assessment forms can be in a standard survey, data collection or checklist format. To demonstrate this process described above, an example of a QA program (plan) will be discussed. Referring to Table 2 the system is Quality Management.

To identify CCPs, ask the question "What are the major/critical processes within this system that must be performed correctly to assure the quality of the finished product/service?" There are ten CCPs listed. Nine of these are cGMP requirements. The tenth CCP, process improvement, has been added to support the concept of "Redefined quality assurance". See Table 3 Quality assurance program (CCPs).

Table 4. Quality Assurance program: System flow chart.

Critical control points	**Application summary**
A through J	Donor suitability
	Blood collection
	Component processing
	Testing
	Review and labelling
	Storage and distribution
	Compatibility testing
	Blood administration
	Investigation of adverse reactions
	Information management

Table 5. Quality Assurance program: Systems.

Quality management CCPs	Donor suitability	Blood collection	Etc.
A. Organizational issues	⇒	⇒	⇒
B. Documentation / Recordkeeping / Record review	⇒	⇒	⇒
Etc.	⇒	⇒	⇒

The KEs for each of these CCPs are then identified. We will take one of the CCPs – Education/training/personnel selection – and list all of the KEs in the next section.

After the CCPs and KEs of the QA program are actually identified, these must be applied across all the other system in blood services. See Tables 4 and 5 Quality assurance program. We will discuss this further when we identify specific KEs, steps leading to the education/training CCP that must be managed to assure error-free processes.

Training for quality assurance

Again QA guidelines are referenced to understand which issues should be addressed. The QA document assigns specific responsibilities to the QA unit in the area of training and education.

1. QA unit will assist in developing, reviewing and ensuring approval of training/educational programs for all manufacturing personnel: recruitment, collections, components, testing, labelling, storage and distribution, MIS and special services.
2. QA unit will ensure tracking capability is available to be used as a management tool
3. QA unit will ensure each employee has a training profile and sign off that employee understands and will cooperate in planning his/her training.
4. QA Unit will ensure the existence of a formal, written annual competency evaluation program which includes direct observation, record review, written tests and, when applicable, use of proficiency samples.
5. QA unit will determine minimum acceptable scores and remedial measures including that employee does not return to work until determined competent by defined process.
6. QA unit will ensure there is a process for reviewing/revising training programs at least annually.
7. QA unit will ensure there is a plan for certifying all trainers.

8. QA unit will ensure that each employee has completed training prior to assuming any duties except in those instances requiring on-the-job training.
9. QA unit will ensure existence of indicators to trigger the need for retraining/training.
10. QA unit will ensure existence of a written plan to evaluate and document effectiveness of training at least annually.
11. QA unit will ensure training program includes the following:
    - New employee orientation
    - cGMP training
    - SOP training/technical training
    - Supervisory/managerial training
    - QA training
    - Computer training
    - Continuing education and training

Not included in the QA guidelines, but critical to the success of implementing a QA program are the following specific types of training:

- Quality awareness training defining the organization's expectation for quality performance.
- Process improvement skills emphasizing the team approach to problem solving.
- Supervisory/management skills to manage teams and facilitate process improvement.

Using the QA guidelines and this additional information the next step in the process is to identify the KEs. KEs are steps leading to the CCPs that must be managed to assure error-free processes. To identify KEs, we ask the question "What are issues that need to be addressed to ensure we are in compliance with all regulations/recommendations?" There are eight KEs for the CCP designated education/training/personnel selection within the quality management system.

Following is a listing of each KE and a short organizational position statement:

1. Position description: Current position descriptions are available for all manufacturing staff.
2. Training profile: Current training profiles describing required training are available for all manufacturing positions.
3. Training format: All training for manufacturing staff conforms to standard training format.
4. Training evaluation: All training programs for manufacturing staff will be appropriately reviewed and evaluated to determine that learning occurred, and to evaluate appropriateness of content, pace, trainer, etc.
5. Training documents and tracking: All training for manufacturing staff requires a system for documentation and a system for tracking.
6. Training competence: A system is in place to assure that all trainers delivering programs relative to manufacturing are competent to deliver approved training programs and to deliver those programs effectively.

7. Training indicators: Key indicators are established and monitored regularly to determine what training/retraining may be necessary for manufacturing staff.
8. Competency evaluation: All manufacturing staff will be certified at least annually, as competent to perform all assigned duties.

The next step in the process described in the QA program section, is to identify the assessment forms to conduct system checks. System checks are the specific activities/tasks to monitor KEs, CCPs and ultimately system function. The following is an example of an assessor's survey suitable for use in assessing the training program:

1. Are materials and programs updated as new processes are implemented?
2. Is this documented?
3. Is training provided before new processes are implemented?
4. Is this documented?
5. Are periodic inservices conducted?
6. Is this documented?
7. Is documentation sufficiently detailed to allow tracking by staff and activity?
8. Are staff with errors/omissions re-trained?
9. Does documentation demonstrate that staff re-training was satisfactorily completed prior to task performance?
10. Is staff trained in the SOPs, cGMPs and other applicable regulations/standards?
11. Does documentation indicate staff is trained and competent to use all equipment?
12. Are staff competent in performance of job tasks?
13. Is this documented?

Having assessed the system, one part of the process described in the QA program is completed. The next activity is to apply each of the CCPs and KEs identified in the QA program (quality management system) to each of the major systems within blood services. That is represented in Tables 4 and 5. For example, we would take each of the KEs within the CCP of education/training personnel selection and assess status in each of the major systems. This next-level assessment can target and prioritize activities and indicate where opportunities for improvement exist.

Using the QA guidelines, we have redefined QA to include QC, cGMP and product assurance. We have described the critical components of the QA program and outlined in detail the KEs of the CCP education/training/personnel selection. This process must be repeated for every system, CCP, KE in the QA program.

Certainly what was the QA concept in 1990 has now been well defined and is being implemented in blood establishments today.

Reference

1. Center for Biologics Evaluation and Research Food and Drug Administration. Draft: Guideline for quality assurance in blood establishments. June 17, 1993. 8800 Rockville Pike Bethesda, Maryland. (Docket No. 91N-0450).

THE GOOD MANUFACTURING PRACTICE CONCEPT

T.F. Zuck

Historical perspective

When *The jungle* was published in 1905 in the United States the general public became aware of the deplorable and filthy conditions in Chicago slaughterhouses [1]. The exposé was written as a social comment about the manner in which the industry treated its employees rather than as an indictment of the unwholesomeness of packed meats. Although deaths caused by consuming infected meat were described, Sinclair's targets were the pitiful living conditions of the workers and their families and the greed of the packing plant owners. The book is widely credited for causing the passage of the Federal Food, Drug and Liquor Act of 1906. The key provision of this act required manufacturers to label their products accurately.

There are parallels in blood banking in the United States today. Through extensive media coverage, public awareness of process control problems in some blood centers has, coupled with the AIDS epidemic, resulted in calls for more vigorous regulation of blood centers. Increased vigour has been generated by the compliance arm of the Food and Drug Administration (FDA) rather than by the professional arm at the center for Biologics Evaluation and Research. The focus of this new emphasis has been upon current Good Manufacturing Practices (cGMP). This focus has significantly changed how blood centers in the United States are regulated.

Biological products were first addressed by an Act of the Congress in 1902. Some key provisions of that act required an establishment license as well as a product license if a product was to be sold legally [2]. The Act also required correct labelling, inspections by designated agents, and suspension, revocation and criminal penalties if the law was violated. These provisions were carried forward to Section 352 of the Public Health Service Act. Both this act and key provisions of regulations issued in 1903 focused on suspension and revocation of licenses as the basic enforcement mechanism, including unannounced inspections [2].

License requirements remain at the heart of FDA's regulatory clout today. As noted, two licenses are required by the Biologics Act of 1902, and they cannot be obtained independently. The establishment license deals with plant, facilities, personnel controls, methods of manufacture, and the like. Section 601.10 of the Code of Federal Regulations (CFR) states explicitly that an establishment license can not be issued unless a "... product license is requested and issued simultaneously with the establishment license." Conversely, Section 602.20 provides that a product license can not be issued "... except upon a determination that the establishment complies with the establishment standards contained in this subchapter..." That is, it has a license. The FDA can use revocation of either license to enforce compliance with the regulation. Thus, if processes for the manufacture of a single product are found wanting, the license for product can be revoked. If an entire product line of an establishment is manufactured with processes not in compliance with the regulations, the establishment license can be suspended or revoked. This recently occurred in the United States to a large manufacturer with a broad product line [3]. Following license suspension, the establishment may no longer ship in interstate commerce any product for sale, barter, or exchange. The FDA may or may not order a recall of products already distributed by a company under license revocation.

An unusual provision of the United States CFR creates an additional regulatory pathway to ensure compliance with the law while relieving the FDA of burdensome inspections. Section 601.22 provides that a licensed establishment may accept partially manufactured products if they are in "short supply" and if the licensed establishment ensures that the shipper is registered and complies with all the regulations related to product safety, purity and potency, that is, cGMP. Human plasma recovered by hospital blood banks has been recognized by the FDA as in short supply. This provision shifts the responsibility from FDA to the licensed establishment to assure that its suppliers are in compliance with cGMP. Shipment by an unlicensed establishment is permitted under what are termed "short-supply agreements" (Section 601.22) in which the shipper agrees to comply with the cGMP provisions of the Code. The licensed establishment has the obligation to assure such compliance.

The Canadian Red Cross recently encountered difficulties with Section 601.22 [Aye R, personal communication, 1993]. Its recovered plasma has been shipped into the United States, custom fractionated by a licensed establishment, and shipped back to Canada for distribution by the Red Cross. The transactions have been conducted under short-supply agreements. Because Canadian centers

Table 1. Examples of early regulatory requirements.*

- Immediate reporting of important establishment changes in personnel, equipment, methods or manufacturing location
- Training and competence of personnel
- Permanent production and control records
- Lot release of some products
- Labelling provisions, including
  - product names
  - expiration dates

* Selected from reference 2.

had not yet brought themselves into compliance with all cGMP requirements, the American fractionator was reluctant to extend the short-supply agreements. Canadian Red Cross centers are becoming compliant in cGMP in order to be able to maintain their fractionation agreements.

Between 1909 and 1919 additional regulations to supplement the Act of 1902 were formulated. Some key provisions are outlined in Table 1. Of particular relevance are requirements for personnel training, production and control records, and reporting important changes in personnel, equipment, or manufacturing methods. The concept of lot release also was introduced in these regulations.

In 1937, an early bactericidal agent, sulfanilamide, was developed into an elixir for pediatric use. Because this compound is essentially insoluble in water, the manufacturer dissolved it in diethylene glycol, an alcohol closely related to antifreeze preparations for automobile radiators. No safety studies were performed and the product was placed on the market. Over a hundred children died before the toxicity of the elixir was appreciated and the product was withdrawn from the market. As with the impact of *The jungle*, this tragedy is believed to have added impetus to the passage of the Food, Drug, and Domestic Act in 1938. Safety became a focus of this legislation. Biologicals were not included in this act, but, as noted earlier, regulatory authority had already been incorporated into Section 352 of the Public Health Service Act.

Thus, the history of the regulation of biological products suggests that the provisions of cGMP are not "new" and they had history spanning over 90 years. It is their strict enforcement in blood centers by cGMP compliance activities that is evolving and perhaps could be described as "new".

cGMP as an industrial concept

cGMP is an industrial rather than a medical concept. This distinction has considerable importance, especially when dealing with blood center processes. Historically, many blood centers have been lead by physicians and industrial concepts were not part of either their training or experience. Yet, the commitment of an organization's leadership becomes a vital component of successful quality improvement based on cGMP concepts. Concerns have been expressed that cGMP implementation in blood centers is not in the best interests of transfusion medicine [4,5]. This debate may be moot, because the regulatory authorities, especially the FDA in the United States, have mandated their implementation in blood centers. But, the concerns of those who oppose cGMP implementation are important. They are particularly important when defining blood center processes. The traditional definitions of medical process have focused on interactions between physicians and patients and health care systems and patients [6]. cGMP and process controls in blood centers are not patient-focused, but rather focused on the interaction of the systems used in the blood centers to manufacture components. In designing cGMP implementation strategies, every effort to mitigate the negative effects voiced by the detractors of implementing cGMP in blood centers should be considered. Some concepts may be useful in addressing their concerns. It has been recommended that blood center management should be organized along functional lines. Traditional medical services, patient consultation, therapeutic apheresis, and the like, should be organizationally separated from the production of blood components [7]. Separating the management of production activities from the management of traditional medical practice permits application of cGMP to the production activities, while permitting the standards of medical practice to define the qualities of medical services. Thus, a blood center addressing the concerns of the loss of professionalism as a result of implementing industrial cGMP models might be structured as diagrammed in Figure 1.

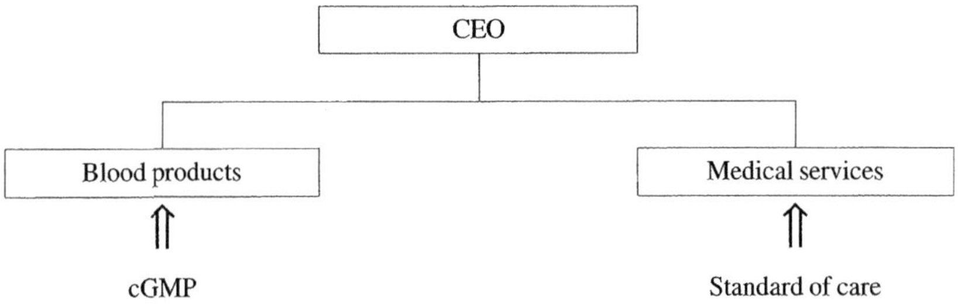

Figure 1. A blood center organizational chart that addresses the need to preserve the practice of transfusion medicine as a center endeavour is illustrated. [See also ref. 7].

As an industrial concept, cGMP echo the current worldwide wave in manufacturing quality improvement. Their basis is simple. In order to improve the quality of what an organization does, process controls should be emphasized rather than the failings of employees [6]. System failure is the cause of most errors, even when those errors were the result of lapses by employees. Because processes are executed by human beings, lapses will occur, and only appropriate process design and control can prevent such lapses from resulting in the release of unsuitable products, in the case of blood banks, components unsuitable for transfusion. FDA inspections based on cGMP precepts ask one question: "Are the processes used to manufacture blood components in this establishment in control?" In this context, 'process' is defined as the sequence of activities that transforms an input, in the case of blood centers, a blood donation, into a final product, in our case blood components [6]. An alternative definition describes a system or a process as a sequence of actions and interactions, between functional units that bring about the manufacture of a product or the delivery of a service [8].

In discussing the controversy about implementing cGMP in blood centers, Miller observed that cGMP will assist them in facing the ever-increasing complexities of running blood centers [9]. In the past decade, blood centers have increased the testing for potential infectious disease transmission from two to eight tests. The challenges of managing the resulting data have similarly increased. cGMP can be viewed as tools or how-to-do roadmaps to the increased demands on blood centers.

Industrial models to achieve quality

Two industrial models have been used to bring about quality improvement. In the traditional detection model, final product testing is used to detect defects. However, Deming taught industry that testing alone would not improve quality, it only describes it [10]. The basis for this conclusion lies in the calculus of errors. If it is assumed that each step in a manufacturing process has a 0.01 per cent failure rate and that there are 1000 steps in manufacturing, the probability of a defective product approaches 10 per cent.The defective product rate can be reduced by decreasing the number of manufacturing steps or decreasing the process error.

But, neither of these steps can be taken without developing process controls that describe the second model, prevention. In the prevention model, quality is achieved by systematically controlling manufacturing processes. Note the similarity here of these concepts to those outlined in the earliest regulations of biologics in 1903.

What, then, are the conceptual cornerstones of the prevention model of industrial quality control as translated into blood center practice by cGMP? That every component released is suitable for transfusion lies at the heart of the concept of lot-to-lot consistency in cGMP. Blood banks have layered their safety protective efforts to guard against an unsuitable release (Table 2). The appropriate management of the individual layers has recently been emphasized by the FDA commissioner [11]. Any error, even if it were detected by a superseding layer and no unsuitable unit were released, is subject to regulatory action. The CFR, then, is both the roadmap for blood centers to comply with cGMP and the regulatory guidelines used by inspectors.

Table 2. cGMP safety layers in blood centers.

– Self-exclusion based on written materials
– Oral donor screening
– Confidential unit exclusion (CUE)*
– After-donation call-back
– Clearance of donor deferral registry
– Hearsay policy
– Donor testing

* CUE is being phased out by most blood centers.

Construct of the cGMP regulations

Section 211 of Title 21 has been referred to as the "umbrella" provision of the cGMP regulations. It not only predates other cGMP provisions, it outlines the fundamental cGMP requirements. Specific provisions for blood banks did not appear in the CFR until 1972, as the series in Sections 606 and 640. It is clearly stated in Section 206.00 that the 200 and 600 series are supplemental to each other and not in lieu of one another. However, it has traditionally been interpreted that if the provision of the two parts of the code are in conflict, the more specific shall. However, if it is possible to comply with all provisions, then compliance is required. Some Sections of the code explicitly state that they do not apply to blood. (See Section 820.1 regarding applicability of medical devices regulations to blood centers).

As a practical matter, one starts to research a problem by consulting Section 211. Having found its provisions, one next turns to 600 Series to determine if more specific provisions may apply and whether they conflict with the provisions of the 200 Series. the general rules stated above apply.

The FDA has tried to clarify how the 200 and 600 Series should be applied to blood centers through a document called the QA guidlines. In its draft form, many difficult areas, such as computer validation and labelling, were left vague and many terms were either poorly defined or left undefined. These deficiencies make their application in day-to-day blood center practice difficult. It is unlikely they will reduce the wide interpretation variances observed during field inspections. Blood centers remain somewhat unclear as to how they are expected to comply with cGMP.

Elements of cGMP

Although not specifically divided as such, the cGMP provisions of the CFR can be separated into elements. This division greatly simplifies both training in and operational applications of cGMP. Table 3 lists one way in which the provisions

Table 3. cGMP elements.

Process controls
Record keeping
Personnel management
Calibration
Validation
Error management
SOPs/Procedures
Labelling
Quality assurance/Audits
Facilities/Equipment

of title 21 can be divided into elements. The meaning of most elements is obvious because their name defines their concept. However, three elements are less obvious and their definitions follows [12].

Validation establishes documented evidence which provides a high degree of certainty that a specific process will consistently produce a product that meets its pre-established quality and performance specifications.

Calibration is the comparison of a measurement standard or instrument of known accuracy with another standard or instrument of unknown accuracy in order to confirm, delete, correlate, report or eliminate by adjustment any variation in the accuracy of the item being compared.

Process control means exercising, restraining or directing influence over the systems used to manufacture components and internally regulating the manner in which these systems function.

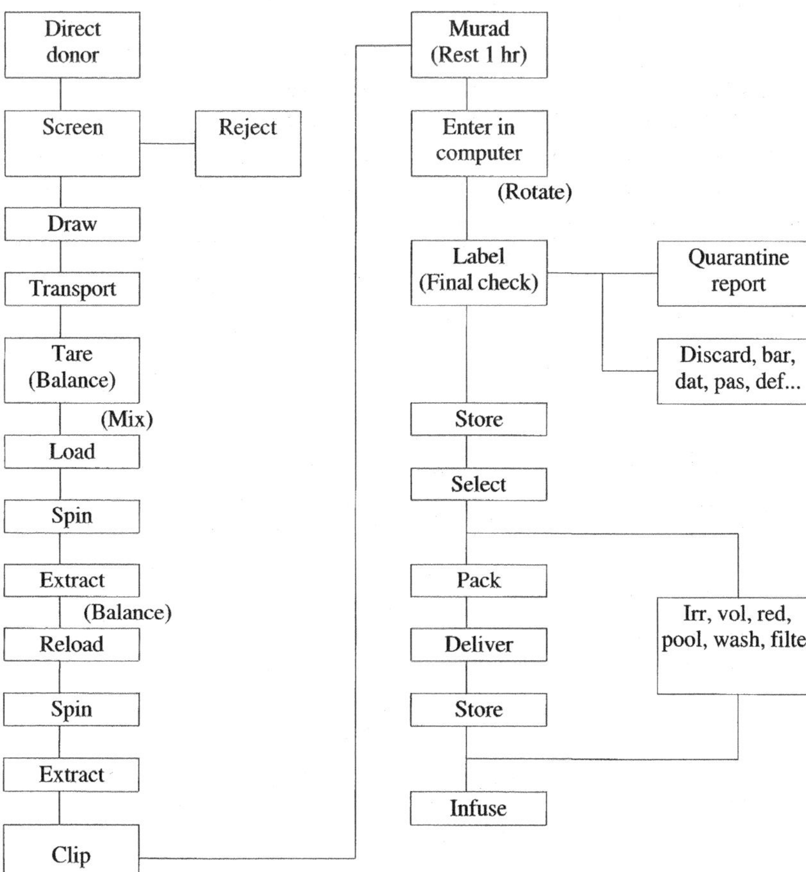

Figure 2. Simplified flow-chart for the manufacture of platelets in a typical blood center is diagramed.

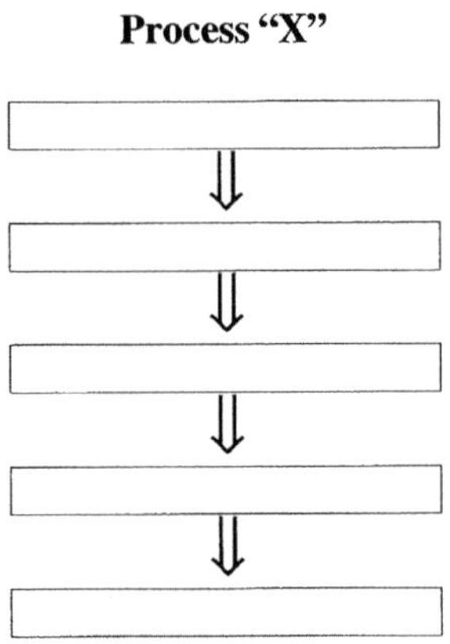

Figure 3. Generic skill-box diagram for any production process in a blood center is shown.

A model of cGMP implementation in blood centers

cGMP implementation can be conceived of having three distinct phases: training, application, and audit. In the first phase, all personnel, from housekeeping staff to the highest ranking manager, must be trained in cGMP as required in Section 211.22.

During the application phase, cGMP elements are applied to all processes used in the manufacture of blood components. This phase is ongoing, for when-

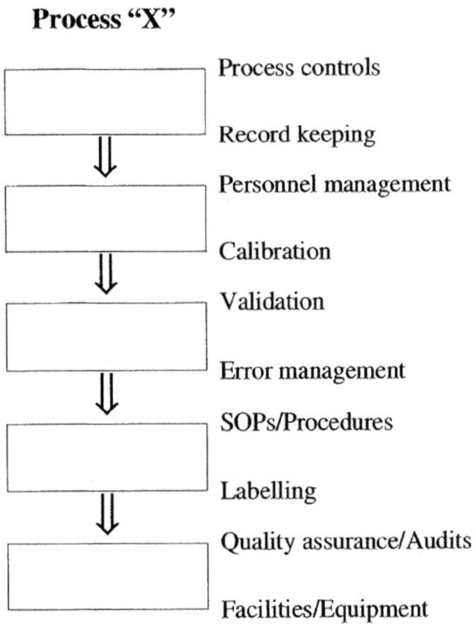

Figure 4. A generic flow-chart with the elements of cGMP listed is diagrammed.

ever a process is changed the elements must again be addressed during the change process. Although many models can be used for this phase, a useful starting place involves process control charting. This activity has many names, but essentially involves developing flow charts for all of the manufacturing processes. In Figure 2, a generalized flow chart is shown for the manufacture of platelets.

A second useful step is to expand the "skill boxes" in the production process diagram. The concept in this exercise is to break down processes to their most basic parts, that is, to a single step in the process. Such a flow diagram for any production process is shown in Figure 3. Each cGMP element can be applied to each of the boxes as illustrated in Figure 4. As an alternative, an element can be applied sequentially to the entire process flow as shown in Figure 5. Either process permits a determination about compliance with cGMP at every step in manufacture. It further permits evaluation of process efficiency. Thus, a determination can be made about whether each of the steps currently in the diagram are essential for manufacture, or if one or more could be consolidated or modified. During this phase, elements found missing must be systematically remedied.

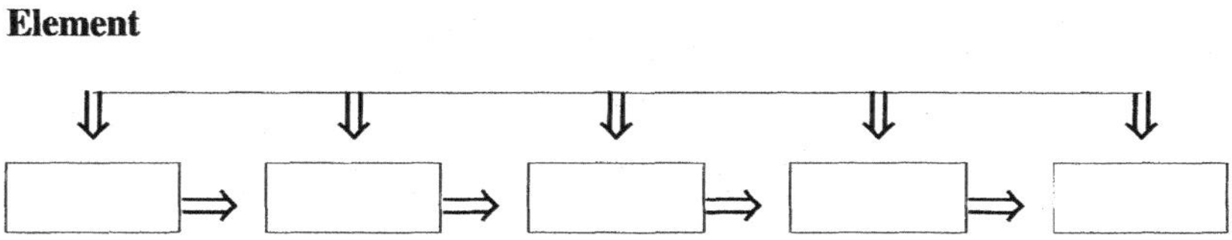

Figure 5. An element is applied vertically to all the skill boxes in a production process in this illustration.

In the third phase of cGMP implementation, the application phase should be audited. That is, did those teams responsible for applying the elements to their processes succeed? Several audit models are available. Commonly, a unit or a group of units is traced through the center to determine the suitability of the manufacturing processes. That activity can be considered a "horizontal audit". As an alternative, a cGMP element could be tracked randomly in manufacturing processes at each level of the organization. This could be termed a "vertical audit". Deficiencies found can be repaired and the corrective action documented.

The three phases of cGMP are completed when corrective action of failures to comply with an element of cGMP is detected during a unit or an element audit. Many blood centers have developed schemes to both perform process engineering on their manufacturing flow and concomitantly implement cGMP. The models proposed in this essay are presented only to illustrate the concepts of cGMP; other models may be equally satisfactory or perhaps superior.

Summary

In this essay, a sense of history for cGMP in the United States is given, emphasizing that the concepts behind cGMP are neither new nor revolutionary. They are designed to assure quality of blood component manufacturing by applying the prevention model of quality control. In this model elements of cGMP are applied to the manufacturing processes in place in the establishment. The cGMP also serve as roadmaps to manage the increasing complexity with which blood centers must cope. Through flow and process diagramming, blood centers can identify each task to which the elements of cGMP apply. The final conceptual piece of cGMP implementation in a center is validation and documentation that a deficiency found in a cGMP audit has been corrected and the remedial action documented.

References

1. Sinclair U. The jungle. Cambridge, MA, Robert Bently, Inc. 1905.
2. Timm EA. 75 Years compliance with biological product regulations. Food Drug Cosmetic Law J 1978;33:225-30.
3. FDA brings injunction against prescription drug manufacturer. CCBC Newsletter. Washington, CCBC, 1993;August 20:1.
4. Polesky HF. Should blood banks institute GMPs? Continues flow. Baxter, Deerfield, IL, 1993;Jan-Feb:4,8.
5. Menitove JE. The recent emphasis on good manufacturing practices and the pharmaceutical manufacturing approach damages blood banking and transfusion medicine as medical care activities. Transfusion 1993;33:439-42.
6. Laffel G, Blumenthal D. The case of using industrial quality management science in health care organizations. JAMA 1989;262:2869-73.
7. Anderson K. Should blood banks institute GMPs? Continuous flow. Baxter, Deerfield, IL, 1993;Jan-Feb:8,10.
8. Kritchevsky SB, Simmons BP. Continuous quality improvement. JAMA 1991;266: 1817-23.
9. Miller WV. Blood banks should use good manufacturing practices and the pharmaceutical manufacturing approach. Transfusion 1993;33:435-8.
10. Deming WE. Out of the crisis. Massachusetts Institute of Technology, Center for Advanced Engineering Study, Cambridge, MA, 1986.
11. Blood manufacturers must act more like drug manufacturers. CCBC Newsletter, Washington, CCBC 1993;July 30:1.
12. Train-the-trainer manual. CCBC and Ortho Diagnostic System, Washington and Raritan 1991.

ERROR POLICIES AND AUDIT SYSTEMS IN TRANSFUSION MEDICINE

K. Sazama

Introduction

About twenty years ago, the Unites States (US) government (through the efforts of the Food and Drug Administration (FDA)) published its regulations (Good Manufacturing Practices, or GMPs) for establishments providing blood components, among which are instructions for handling "errors and accidents" [1]. A curious omission from these regulations is the lack of definition of either "error" or "accident". No further clarification of the intended meaning of these two terms has been made by the US government in any subsequently published guidance.

Using Merriam-Webster's 1993 Collegiate Dictionary, 10th edition [2], several definitions for both "error" and "accident" can be found (Tables 1 and 2). With no single definition provided from de FDA to provide clarification, any or all may be assumed to be applicable. Also, something important can be appreciated from these definitions. Both terms encompass the ideas of no intent and of insufficient knowledge or ignorance leading to harm or injury. If accidents and

Table 1. An error is any of the following acts or conditions.

- Ignorant or imprudent deviation from a code of behaviour.
- An unintentional deviation from truth or accuracy.
- Through ignorance, deficiency, or accident, departing from or failing to achieve what should be done.
- A mistake in the proceedings of a court of record in matters of law or of fact.

Table 2. An accident is

- An unforeseen and unplanned event or circumstance occurring with lack of intention or necessity.
- An unfortunate event resulting especially from carelessness or ignorance.
- An unexpected and medically important bodily event, especially when injurious.
- An unexpected happening causing loss or injury which is not due to any fault or misconduct on the part of the person injured but for which legal relief may be sought.

Accidents are "not amenable to planning or prediction", and are chance events.

Table 3. An audit is

- A formal examination of an organization's or individual's accounts or financial situation.
- A methodical examination and review.

Table 4. Error rates for transfusion.

Date	Author	Number of transfusions	Error rate
1959	Binder [8]	81,392	1 in 2700
1963	Schmidt [10]	5,806	1 in 100
1966	Kwa [11]		1 in 2000
1972	Lacerte [12]		1 in 3
1974	Taswell [13]	62,590	1 in 500
1984	Taswell [14]		1 in 100 to 1 in 1000
1992	Linden [15]	1,784,600	1/19,000

errors are unintended and unforeseen, then responses to them should emphasize changing human behaviour [3] but should focus instead on identifying and correcting system flaws [4] (only in some instances when either error or accident occurs through carelessness or dereliction would efforts to change human behaviour be appropriate). However, because even now the words "error", "accident" and "audit" (Table 3) lack standard definition, published error reports lack comparability from institution to institution (Table 4). Perhaps the most consistent application of a single definition has been that of Taswell who has uniformly defined an error as "an inadvertent or unauthorized deviation from standard procedure" [5].

Focus on human error

The ultimate error in blood transfusion is fatality directly caused by the transfused component, virtually always attributable to human error. As late as 1956, ABO incompatible transfusions occurred with an incidence of 0.7% and mortality rates as high as 25% [6]. However, although overall risks of transfusion-associated fatality as high as 1/13,000 in Great Britain [7], and 1/11,000 in the US [8] have been reported in recent years, in the 1990s this risk in the US is probably closer to 1/250,000 [9].

To address this problem in 1953, a "... simple yet rigid system of check, check, and counter-check ..." was recommended in which only physicians were permitted to remove blood from the cold storage area and actually administer it to patients, with a second person (often a nurse) witnessing the event [7]. As recently as 1989, Australian transfusionists were advised "... to shift emphasis ... to the strict following of standard established protocols for transfusion ... to minimize the possibility of (ABO) accidents due to human error" [16].

For a number of years internal institutional review of transfusion practices has been advocated by US accrediting organizations such as the Joint Commission on Accreditation of Healthcare Organizations, the American Association of Blood Banks, and the College of American Pathologists as well as by transfusion medicine specialists. These internal, periodic systematic investigations to confirm or negate that established, approved policies and SOPs are being properly implemented ("internal audits") are used to evaluate appropriateness of component use and to avoid or minimize adverse reactions [17]. A significant omission from such reviews may be that there are no standards to evaluate *under*transfusion of patients whose clinical status would justify such intervention [18]. Even with such routine systems of error detection, Brodheim estimated that in 1988 there was "... one error associated with every 10 to 20 blood components transfused" [19].

The longitudinal study of errors from which the most comprehensive data are available from the Mayo Clinics where error detection systems have been in use for more than ten years [20]. Using an error classification system based on function, Taswell et al. have found interesting patterns of error reduction in identification, performance, transcription, interpretation and storage and retrieval with appropriate changes in systems over this time frame [20]. Smit Sibinga using this same approach found that "performance is by far the most frequently occurring functional type of (error)" [21]. Other published systems for detection and assessment of errors and accidents range from informal recognition and interception [10] and formal periodic audits [17,22,23] (including selfinspections) to external inspections and even deliberate introduction of errors into routine work practices [24]. Error preventing efforts in transfusion services may now include not only auditing actual transfusion events [25], but also performing delta checks to detect sample mistakes [26-28], evaluating arrangements of blood components in refrigerated storage [29], surveying practices nationally [30,31] and conducting ongoing reviews of well-defined processes [32].

Nearly all error detection/prevention efforts are focused on changing human behaviour [33] rather than improving systems, even though as long ago as 1958, Binder commented that "The persistence of the *same* human errors in the *same* order of frequency in spite of extensive efforts to eradicate them also suggests their *inherent irreducible quality*" [8]. Three decades later, Taswell agrees, stating "Since it is not reasonable to expect human error to occur with a frequency of less than 1/10,000, the only way to improve ... is by making major system changes." [14].

Systems approach to error reduction

While innovative approaches to improvement of routine transfusion practices are still uncommon [34], the value of a systems correction approach to blood banking errors has been well documented over time at the Mayo Clinics (Figure 1). Introduction of a computerized reporting and filling system reduced errors tenfold in their facility (Figure 2). Their "closed-loop" organization that can control

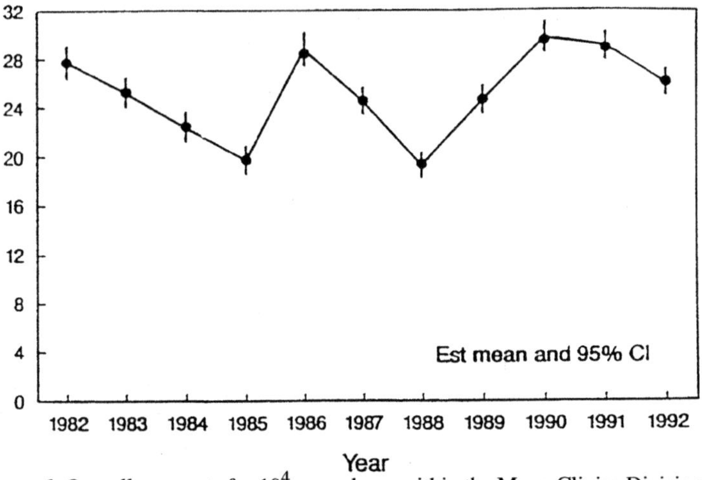

Figure 1. Overall error rate for 10^4 procedures within the Mayo Clinics Division of Transfusion Medicine [from ref. 32].

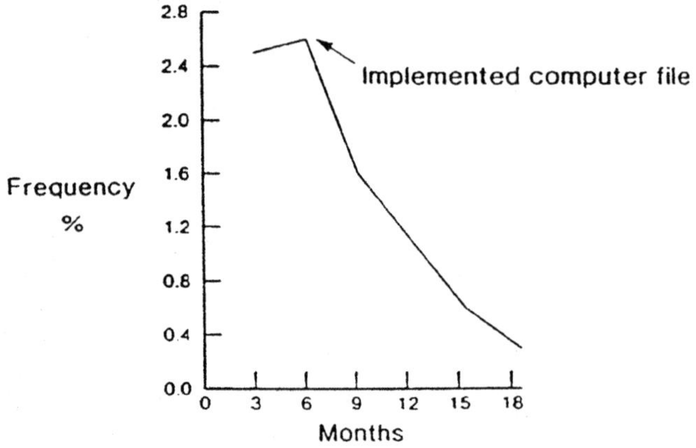

Figure 2. Change in error rate following implementation of a computer file for storage and retrieval of patient information in the Mayo Clinics Division of Transfusion Medicine [from ref. 14].

all aspects of transfusion, from collection through infusion, permits their regular comprehensive audit and review of practices, including use of quantitative data for error reduction [35,36].

Another example of the value of a systems approach is that from an American Red Cross blood collection center which reduced one source of error, blood labelling, by 80% (from 35/million units to @7/million units) through use of an automated system comparing current ABO results against previous results from repeat blood donors [37].

Rigorous analyses of laboratory errors, particularly from clinical chemistry laboratories, where overall error rates of 3 [38] to 3.5% [39] led to the recognition in 1972 of the necessity for "undertak(ing) a program of systematic improvement of laboratory performance" [39], have encouraged widespread use of automation, with bar coding of specimens now in routine use in many such laboratories [40].

However, a recently published report of 9% *analytical* error rate in laboratories, undetectable by "customary" QC/QA methods [41], is surprising in light of the continuing efforts undertaken by manufacturers and laboratorians to minimize or eradicate such errors. Robotics replacement of human actions for numerous routine laboratory functions has and hopefully will continue to reduce error rates [42].

Emphasis on prevention in quality management policies

A major problem with most approaches to errors (even the system used by the Mayo Clinics studies) is their routine dependence upon recognition of a mistake *after its occurrence* [43,44]. Recent US regulatory guidance stresses the need to not only identify and correct errors as or after they occur, but also a more general interest in avoiding commission of such mistakes altogether. Newer concepts of quality assurance, including the language in the US FDA's newest guideline on QA [45], encompass the requirement for prospective intervention to prevent errors from occurring. The process now required by the FDA is shown in Tables 5 and 6.

Systems targeted for error prevention within modern transfusion practice may benefit from personal intervention, as demonstrated by Shulman and colleagues who effected 100% compliance with existing transfusion administration procedures [46] (Figure 3). An understanding of estimates of current (1992) average rates of error which in the US is thought to be between 20 to 30/10,000 procedures (including errors overall, by area of activity and by type of function) [32], or looking at how to minimize the impact of sample swapping [47] and misidentification of patients [48] as well as introducing standards to prevent *under*-transfusion as well as reducing unnecessary transfusions in some clinical settings [49] are other areas in which intervention can be applied successfully.

Table 5. Conducting internal audits.

- Planned and periodic reviews.
- Conducted via SOP specifying procedure.
- Defined in purpose and scope.
- Checklist.
- Personnel-trained, analytical, no direct responsibility.
- Scheduled initiation and completion.

Table 6. Records or internal audits

- Operation or function.
- Responsible head.
- Identity of auditor.
- Full report of findings.
- Corrective actions recommended.
- Schedule for repeat audit.
- Recommendations for general improvements.

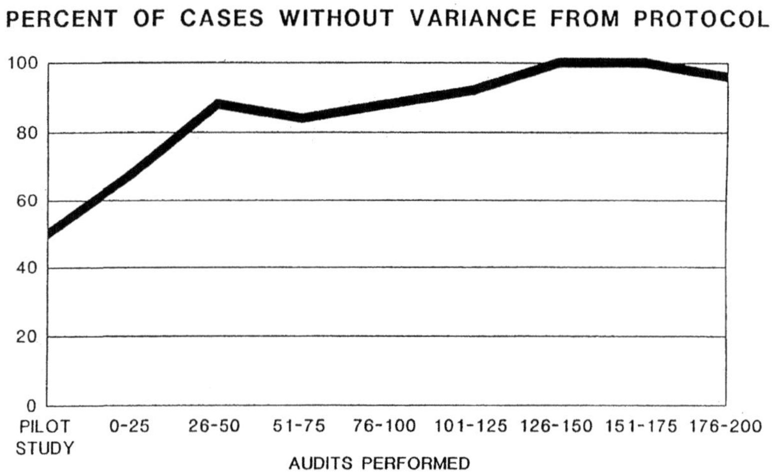

Figure 3. Performance improvement by targeted audits in LAC/USC Division of Transfusion Medicine [from ref. 42].

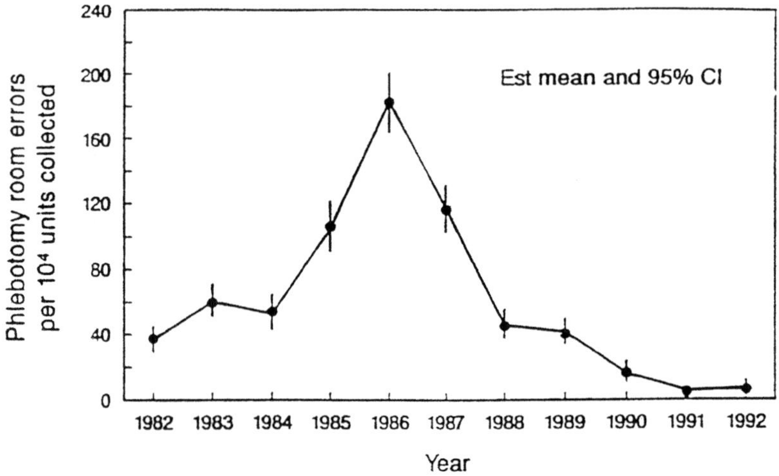

Figure 4. Performance errors per 10^4 units collected in the phlebotomy room in the Mayo Clinic Division of Transfusion Medicine [from ref. 32].

An important aspect hidden within these new guidelines is that the action of making changes within systems may *introduce* errors, at least temporarily. These new FDA QA guidelines may fail to take into account the adverse effect that introduction of necessary changes into an existing system can have, including the actual increase in errors initially as shown in Figure 1 from the Mayo Clinics experience. Part of this increase in errors at the Mayo Clinics coincided with introduction of the commonality label in 1986. The number of errors in the Mayo Clinics phlebotomy area tripled initially, but declined to consistently lower error levels over subsequent years (Figure 4). Thus, short term effects of changing systems should be evaluated with caution, recognizing the inevitable perturbations inherent in such events. The US FDA commissioner, David Kessler, who has expressed dismay at the speed of changes within the US blood banking "industry" [50], may have an unrealistic expectation of outcomes demanded of blood banks when considering the number of changes required. The longer term benefits of improvements should be anticipated and measured appropriately, including reasonable understanding and acceptance of predictable momentary variations in error rates as change is introduced into existing systems.

Conclusions

Evaluation of errors within blood collection and transfusion facilities requires strict definition of errors with uniform application of terms to the systems analysis required. When change occurs as rapidly as has been the case during the 1980s and early 1990s, introduction of new instruments, procedures, technologies (including computerization) and personnel requirements carry an implicit opportunity for an *initial* transient increase in error rates, followed by a decline to lower levels than prior to the change. This predictable "blip" of adjustment may be (and apparently often is) misinterpreted as lack of positive outcome from required changes when inspections by accrediting and regulating agencies occur too frequently. Better data collected using a generally accepted definition of the terms "errors" and "accidents" should provide a firm basis for prudent evaluations and assessments. The Mayo Clinics and Red Cross Blood Bank Groningen-Drenthe experiences are one solid example of such a system, with proven benefits of its use.

References

1. Title 21, Code of Federal Regulations, §600.10, US Government Printing Office, current edition.
2. Merriam-Webster's Collegiate Dictionary, 10th Edition, Springfield, MA, 1993.
3. Sherwood WC. To err is human ... Transfusion 1990;30:579-80.
4. Sazama K. Reports of 355 transfusion-associated deaths: 1976 through 1985. Transfusion 1990;30:583-90.
5. Taswell F. The philosophy of quality assurance in the blood bank. In: Quality assurance in blood banking and its clinical impact. (Smit Sibinga CTh, Das PC, Taswell HF (eds). Martinus Nijhoff Publishers, Boston, 1984:XI-XIII.

6. Hall JE, Hellman LM. Transfusion reactions in obstetrics Obstet Gynecol 1957;9: 250-7.
7. Blood transfusion accidents. Br Med J 1953;2:390-1.
8. Binder LS, Ginsberg V, Harmel MH. A six year study of incompatible blood transfusions. Surg Gynecol Obstet 1959;108:19-34.
9. Consensus Development Panel, National Institutes of Health. Perioperative red blood cell transfusion. JAMA 1988;260:2700-3.
10. Schmidt PJ, Kevy SV. Sources of error in a hospital blood bank. Transfusion 1963;3:198-201.
11. Kwa SB, Ariff KB. Blood banking errors: A two year prospective survey. Singapore Med J 1966;7:178-84.
12. Lacerte JM, Kane VM, Cohen P. US licensed blood banks: Evaluation of whole blood and its components. Transfusion 1972;12:339-43.
13. Taswell HF, Smith AM, Sweat MA, Pfaff KJ. Quality control in the blood bank: A new approach. Am J Clin Pathol 1974;62:491-5.
14. Taswell HF, Sonnenberg CL. Error analysis: Types of errors in the blood bank. In: Quality assurance in blood banking and its clinical impact. Smit Sibinga CTh, Das PC, Taswell HF (eds). Martinus Nijhoff Publishers, Hingham, MA, 1984:227-37.
15. Linden JV, Paul B, Dressler KP. A report of 104 transfusion errors in New York State. Transfusion 1992;32:601-6.
16. Bacon JM, Young IF. ABO incompatible blood transfusion. Pathology 1989;21:181-4.
17. Silberstein LE, Kruskall MS, Stehling LC, et al. Strategies for the review of transfusion practices. JAMA 1989;262:1993-7.
18. Lenfant C. Audit for undertransfusion as well as for overuse of blood components. Qual Rev Bull 1992;18:214.
19. Brodheim E. The role of automatic identification methods and techniques in blood transfusion. In: Automation in blood transfusion. Smit Sibinga CTh, Das PC, Högman CF (eds). Kluwer Academic Publishers, Boston, 1988:9-21.
20. Sonnenberg CL, Taswell HF. Error analysis: Methods of detection, analysis and control. In: Quality assurance in blood banking and its clinical impact. Smit Sibinga CTh, Das PC, Taswell HF (eds). Martinus Nijhoff Publishers, Boston, 1984:239-46.
21. Smit Sibinga CTh, Thie JH, Smit Z. Quarantine control and release of blood and blood components. In: Automation in blood transfusion. Smit Sibinga CTh, Das PC, Högman CF (eds). Kluwer Academic Publishers, Boston, 1988:153-61.
22. Simpsom MB. Audit criteria for transfusion practices. In: The hospital transfusion committee. Wallas CH, Muller VH (eds). American Association of Blood Banks, Arlington, VA, 1982:21-58.
23. Nicholls MD. Quality assurance of hospital transfusion practice. Med J Aust 1993;158:295-7.
24. Taswell HF, Smith AM, Sweatt MA, Pfaff KJ. Quality control in the blood bank: A new approach. Am J Clin Pathol 1974;62:491-5.
25. Murphy WG, McClelland DBL. Deceptively low morbidity from failure to practice safe blood transfusion: An analysis of serious blood transfusion errors. Vox Sang 1989;57:59-62.
26. Nosanchuk JS, Gottman AW. CUMS and delta checks: A systematic approach to quality control. Am J clin Pathol 1974;62:707-12.
27. Sheiner LB, Wheeler LA, Moore JK. The performance of delta check methods. Clin Chem 1979;25:2034-7.
28. Iizuka Y, Kume H, Kitamura M. Multivariate delta check method for detecting specimen mix-up. Clin Chem 1982;28:2244-8.
29. Shulman IA, Kent D. Unit placement errors, a potential risk factor for ABO and Rh incompatible blood transfusions. Lab Med 1991;22:194-6.
30. Levy GJ, Strauss RG, Hume H, et al. National survey of neonatal transfusion practices. I. Red blood cell therapy. Pediatr 1993;91:423-529.

31. Strauss RG, Levy GJ, Sotelo-Avila C, et al. National survey of neonatal transfusion practices. II. Blood component therapy. Pediatr 1993;91:530-6.
32. Taswell H, Galbreath JL, Harmsen WS. Errors in transfusion medicine: Detection, analysis, frequency and prevention. Arch Pathol Lab Med 1994 (in press).
33. Sharp DE, Cook SS, Gervin AS. Transfusion related mortalities: Prior lessons unlearned. Transfusion 1984;24:433. Abstract.
34. Wenz B, Burns ER. Improvement in transfusion safety using a new blood unit and patient identification system as part of safe transfusion practice. Transfusion 1991;31: 401-3.
35. Taswell HF, Watts SK, Downie CM, DeBusman G. A closed-loop identification system for blood bank processes. Transfusion 1985;25:496.
36. Taswell HF, Grosset J, Meine D, DeBusman G. Automation in transfusion practice: Storage and retrieval of transfusion information. In: Automation in blood transfusion. Smit Sibinga CTh, Das PC, Högman CF (eds). Kluwer Academic Publishers, Boston, 1988:193-200.
37. Grindon AJ, Liles BA. Center error reduction by recheck of blood type. Transfusion 1981;21:199.
38. McSwiney RR, Woodrow DA. Types of errors within a clinical laboratory. J Med Lab Technol 1969;26:340-6.
39. Grannis GF, Gruemer H-D, Lott JA, Edison JA, McCabe WC. Proficiency evaluation of clinical chemistry laboratories. Clin Chem 1972;18:222-36.
40. Whisler K, Maffeton M, Watt S. Automated system for positive specimen identification and sample handling. Clin Chem 1990;36:1587-8.
41. Kazmierczak SC, Catrou PG. Laboratory error undetectable by customary quality control/quality assurance monitors. Arch Pathol Lab Med 1993;117:714-8.
42. DeMoranville VE, Ellis JE. Examples of enhanced laboratory workflow through the application of robotics. Clin Chem 1990;36:1588-90.
43. Blanchette VS, Hume HA, Levy GJ, Luban NLC, Strauss RG. Guidelines for auditing pediatric blood transfusion practices. Am J Dis Child 1991;145:787-96.
44. Hoeltge GA, Brown JC, Herzig RH, et al. Computer-assisted audits of blood component transfusion. Cleveland Clinic J Med 1989;56:267-72.
45. Guideline for quality assurance in blood establishments. US Food and Drug Administration, June 17, 1993.
46. Shulman IA, Lohr K, Derdiaria AK, Picukaric JM. Monitoring transfusionist practices, a strategy for improving transfusion safety. Transfusion 1994;34:11-5.
47. Soloway HB, Kaplan HS. Mathematical implications of inadvertent sample swapping and the preception of apparent rates of gross error. Clin Chem 1990;36:1525-6.
48. Renner SW, Howantiz PJ, Bachner P. Wristband identification error reporting in 712 hospitals. Arch Pathol Lab Med 1993;117:573-7.
49. Meyer J, Sive A, Jacobs P. Empiric red cell transfusion in asymptomatic preterm infants. Acta Paediatr 1993;82:30-4.
50. FDA slams blood banking industry. Advance for Medical Laboratory Professionals, 1993;August 23:5,14.

DISCUSSION

H.J. Heiniger and H.I. Hannema

H. Bremer (Eindhoven, NL): Looking to the vocabulary I think it is very important to use wording that one understands. Definitions are not always easy and I remember a meeting some time ago when I was sitting with Canadians, Americans, Welshmen and Scotsmen to arrive at a definition of terms such as "audit" and "assessment". It took us six hours! Nevertheless, deliberations like this have led to agreement and I draw your attention to ISO-TC176 Definitions and Terms as laid down in document ISO 8402. Work is continuing and this "dictionary" is being developed for worldwide use.

C.Th. Smit Sibinga (Groningen, NL): Just to take away any mis-conception: I am well aware of the ISO vocabulary in this respect.

H.J. Heiniger (Bern, CH): I have a question regarding the audit. Do you include in "inadvertently" also a lack of training?

C.Th. Smit Sibinga: Yes indeed, because if there is a lack of training one has assigned the wrong responsibilities to a person, based on a lack of training to not being able really carry out what is expected. That is an error at a different level. You cannot blame the person for that, you should blame the organization.

H.J. Heiniger: Dr. Robins, could you give us an idea what this new effort as compared to the old Quality Control (QC) effort means in percentage of cost increase for an institution. What do you estimate?

J.L. Robins (New York, NY, USA): We talk about this in terms of price per product. I think, certainly in the beginning, our estimates are that we are adding approximately a dollar per product. That may seem a lot, but that is an initial investment. I am sure mr. Bremer would agree, as we put all these process improvements and activities, and giving people tools to do their job better in place, we hope to see productivity gains. We hope to rid our processes of the waste and rework any time an error is made. If you have to correct that error if it goes out of the blood centre, there are untold dollars. It is hard to calculate how much time we spend on reportable errors in the United States. The Quality Assurance (QA) movement has not yet really put its arms around how to calculate the cost of quality. The benefit is certainly going to counterbalance. All QA costs we expect will generate saving in the future.

A. Heaton (San Francisco, CA, USA): Ms. Robins, how many employees does the non-plasma side of your blood program have and how many employees do you have involved in QA.

J.L. Robins: Can I give you the number of products we distribute a year and tell you our staff ratio?

A. Heaton: I would prefer to know the ratio of quality assurance employees to the total employees.

J.L. Robins: We have 1200 employees in our blood center in the blood services and we have 19 people in the quality department. We distribute 1.5 million products a year.

H.J. Heiniger: Dr. Zuck, since these guidelines, were as you said, formulated at the turn of the century, why do you think they only became really burning in the last ten years.

T.F. Zuck (Cincinnati, OH, USA): Four letter word? – AIDS.

At least in the United States, the public has enormous concern about the transmission of AIDS and then they became concerned about other transmissible diseases. I do not think it is that much different in Europe than in the United States. In France as you know, the hemophiliacs really pressed the issue in the news and electronic media, and jail terms resulted. So, everybody got terrified. We respond to being terrified in a political way by legislatures and by the Food and Drug Administration. Blood centers responded because they really did understand that some of our systems were not optimal and we went back and looked at things. So I think two things happened: AIDS brought on a public reaction and a private response.

H.J. Heiniger: However, before this there was also hepatitis, but this did not trigger by far a similar reaction.

T.F. Zuck: There is not the same emotional attachment or fear of hepatitis as there is for AIDS. It may not be reasonable, but it is true.

J. Szabo (Budapest, H): Dr. Zuck, do you circulate a deferral list of the donors amongst the blood banks?

T.F. Zuck: The answer to your question in the short term is no we do not. We are the only blood center in our community. So, to send a list to other hospitals would not be of any practical value. There has been a significant discussion in the United States about whether a national registry of a country our size and the mobility in our country would be worth pursuing. There are some political forces that want to see it happen and also analysis of the data about the efficiency of such a system. You will find out that a national system would intercept very few donors in the United States based on how our system operates.

Dr. Sazama, I do not have a definition for urgent, but I am going to ask you a question. The FDA has defined something that is reportable as an error or an accident that makes a component available for transfusion. I understand that it is not perfect, but I think it gives some clarification. You did not mention it, is there some reason that you think this is an adequate definition?

K. Sazama (Sacramento, CA, USA): Yes, the example I gave of bacterial contamination is one of those that we need to think carefully about. Inherent in the definitions of both error and accident is that it is something beyond the control of human performance. The raw material from which we obtain the product to be transfused is human. If the error occurs due to human-human interaction, what kind of a system change would be effective? In terms of the particular problem of bacterial contamination, when it has been traced, the conclusion has been that there was no way it could have been predicted. From most of the circumstances, it would have been the inevitable consequence. So, one way to handle errors is to try to emphasize that it is important to know what the definitions are and to be consistent with those definitions.

T.F. Zuck: Well, that would fall into the generic rule. If you know that a recipient became infected, without regard for determining cause, you released or made available for release something unsuitable for transfusion. The importance of reporting it clearly is, that it might be a lot of bags that might have been infected. If FDA gets three reports of that same lot, it would mean a recall.

K. Sazama: I completely agree with what you are saying. If the source of the contamination is not from the human donor, but rather from some other flaw in the system, that is a reason why it should be reported. I was trying to illustrate the point that it may be by virtue of neither an error nor an accident that the product is unsafe. It is extremely important that we be rigorous regarding what it is we intend to report.

I. Helsper (Utrecht, NL): Will it help to use the term non-conformance instead of error, because you could define non-conformance as a deviation to any authorized document like a specification.

K. Sazama: That term has some appeal. It also removes any sort of psychological overlay with a periorative connotation that both "error" or "accident" suggests that somebody could have done something about it. If the product comes up in "non-conformance", then you can focus your corrective efforts properly.

D.B.L. McClelland (Edinburgh, UK): Mr. Bremer, I enjoyed your talk immensely. I wonder if you or anyone on the panel would comment on the proposition that the further development of very strictly drawn regulatory standards is totally inimical to the concept of people-driven continuous quality improvement. It seems to me the reconciliation between these two issues is a major problem.

H. Bremer: I think you are right, at least if we go further along the Taylor way and develop more standards. Such standards would force us to have more inspections and more audits. That is contrary to people-oriented TQM. For your information, in ISO we realize that that is not the way to go. Just recently a task force was established to develop a guide for a generic management system, people-oriented TQM based. From there on we will develop standards, which will fit into that way of thinking. That will, however, take quite some years, perhaps not until 2002. However, by approximately 1997, ISO will issue a new set of standards replacing the current ISO 9000 and 10,000 series. These will be somewhere in between.

A. Heaton: As one looks at a processing system for manufacturing product, it is common practice to start with a set of product specifications. One of the issues that I would like to discuss with the panel is the fact that in manufacturing blood there are no product specifications. In practice we have only donor specifications, in that we only know what our minimum hematocrit must be and also the minimum quantity of blood withdrawn. What this means is that we do not have final product specifications for a unit of red cells. Do you think we should in fact develop true product specifications and minimum product standards?

H. Bremer: Well, as you know I am more or less educated in industry. Usually one starts with defining product specifications before products will be developed and produced.

T.F. Zuck: One of the fundamental differences between the CFR 200 series and the CFR 600 series is that we have very little control over the raw material from which we are processing. It is very interesting that if you have a manufacturing plant, there are very rigid controls and qualifications when it brings in raw materials. There will be all kinds of testing procedures to qualify materials to be manufactured further. We do not have that and we cannot have that. But one of the recognitions between CFR 200 and CFR 600 for us is to test the product rigidly. In an alternative you try to control the manufacturing process for cGMP and lot-to-lot variation.

C.Th. Smit Sibinga: Actually, dr. Heaton, in our country we decided through the mechanism of the National Council of Blood Transfusion to draft in consensus and put in place guidelines on specifications of blood products for the sake of coming to at least minimum acceptable standards in the manufacturing, the quality control, in the release and ultimately providing to the clinic specified blood products. I would be happy to share those guidelines with you.

A. Heaton: I am very interested in this and I feel that we probably should devote more effort towards developing product specifications. We have an analysis of product specifications under review for the International Forum Section in Vox Sanguinis,[1] where we have attempted to statistically identify the sample size that one would need to measure in order to correctly identify deviation from product specifications. At the moment in the US, we only have a requirement to test four platelet concentrates a month, which is meaningless given component productions rates which may exceed 1000 a week.

C.Th. Smit Sibinga: The minimum acceptable sampling size is in these specifications guideline. I will share that with you.

H.J. Heiniger: Just a comment. The Committee of Quality Control of the Council of Europe also has drafted guidelines for these specifications. They may be as dr. Smit Sibinga said minimum requirements and definitions, which may be revised. These guidelines are available from the Council of Europe.

T.F. Zuck: I would like to respond to the European approach. It is very true that the four platelets the FDA requires is a joke. You can count thousands, which we have done with the help of the engineering school, to develop the statistical process. If you do it, you can get larger sampling sizes and thereby increase the statistical power. You still are stuck with the problem that the FDA defines a lot or batch as one bag of something. In industry you test a batch by sampling the batch. You cannot do that practically with blood and blood components. I completely agree with my European peers that you can increase the statistical power by counting more but you still have not released the batch. That is the problem.

D.B.L. McClelland: Can I come back to dr. Heaton's question? To be a little provocative, it seems to me to be completely crazy to be worrying about the fine detail of the specification of a red cell unit. If you look at what you achieve within for example the United Kingdom's standard specifications, the unit can have anywhere between a 150 and 220 ml of red cells in it. You give the product to the clinician as a bag of oxygen carrying and delivering medium. I think we need to go back to the problem design first and then make the specification.

1. Definitions, which may be revised. These guidelines are available from the Council of Europe.

B.T. Teague (Houston, TX, USA): Mr. Bremer and the panel, I would like your definition of safe and then I would like to hear from the blood bankers their definition of safe.

K. Sazama: In the United States, the words "safe" and "blood transfusion" have become and oxymoronic. The perception of what is safe is yet to be further defined. Certainly the patients who find themselves unexpectedly the recipients of something they believed would be life-saving which in fact has the ultimate opposite effect would never agree with any definition that we, who collect and transfuse blood, would apply. So, the definition of "safe" in the United States with respect to blood is very problematic.

M. McGregor (Cardiff, UK): Mr. Bremer, since ISO have produced a standard for quality management systems, surely what the international transfusion world should be looking for is their interpretation of the elements of the standards rather than every country going around producing their own management system.

H. Bremer: Thank you very much for this remark. What we see now in most parts of the world is that people start to understand that massive and expensive inspections can, for the greater part, effectively be replaced by Quality Systems (QS). The next step is that those people start to develop their "own" QS, in most cases simply because they do not know that the ISO material is already available. Others think that ISO standards cannot be applied in their field of operation, because of the "we are different" syndrome. As I see it, if a branch (e.g. blood banks worldwide) wish to develop a series of QA standards in their own "language", the present ISO standards should/must be used as source documents in order to prevent a worldwide proliferation of standards and associated practices. This means that the contents should be fully in line with the ISO standards,

Table 1. GMP in transfusion medicine.

Total quality management (TQM) NEN-ISO 8402: Quality systems. Vocabulary NEN-ISO 9000/EN 29000 series
– NEN-ISO 9000/EN 29000 Quality management and quality assurance standards: Guidelines for selection and use
– NEN-ISO 9001/EN 29001 Quality systems: Model for quality assurance in design/development, production, installation and service
– NEN-ISO 9002/EN 29002 Quality systems: Model for quality assurance in production and installation
– NEN-ISO 9003/EN 29003 Quality systems: Model for quality assurance in final inspection and test
– NEN-ISO 9004/EN 29004 Quality management and quality system elements: Guidelines

though the vocabulary could be adapted to the branch. The present Quality Management (QM) standard (ISO 9004) will shortly be replaced by an updated version. As I said before, within ISO, a task force has been set up recently to develop a new document regarding Generic Management Systems.

C.Th. Smit Sibinga: To the blood banking community and anyhow to the medical community the ISO set of standards and recommendations is not very well known. The main themes of the various parts of the ISO regulations are presented in Table 1. This is basically the essence and they are really of importance also to our blood transfusion world.

H. Bremer: Can I add to this. These are the basic documents, but there are many more. Vocabulary, how to write a quality manual, organize all your paperwork and so on, guidelines and also standards. They are all available.

K. Sazama: I would like to direct this question to dr. Robins and, perhaps, to dr. Zuck. I wonder if you can share with us how much of your original efforts for quality improvement of processes were devoted to establishing a baseline against which future comparisons would be made, especially with respect to establishing existing error levels for common parameters.

J.L. Robins: In the beginning we decided that, what we did the first three months should become our baseline, because we felt that people were still learning. We did not try to go back, we did not try to resurrect or recreate. So whatever came out of the first three months became our baseline.

T.F. Zuck: We decided to measure through an existing program with continuous improvement of error management. When we started on the program the number of errors that were reported increased absolutely beyond our wildest expectations, because people were looking for them and there was no punity for having found them. In fact, they were given credits for having reported them. Then it settled back down to roughly what it was before and now it has dropped below it was. We just used the error reporting as a tool.

D.B.L. McClelland: Can I ask dr. Sazama to expand on one point. You said in your presentation that the true rate of ABO related fatalities was approximately tenfold higher than the figures that you showed. I am very interested in that.

K. Sazama: Let me just correct that impression. If I have stated that tenfold rate as applying only to ABO errors, that is a mistake. My comment was intended to convey that there is a possibly tenfold underreporting rate for all fatalities from transfusion. The more specific evidence for this underreporting is based on reviewing a number of reports of graft-versus-host disease fatalities from transfusion. Just scanning the English language literature for reports of transfusion-induced GvHD fatalities reported only by institutions subject to US FDA

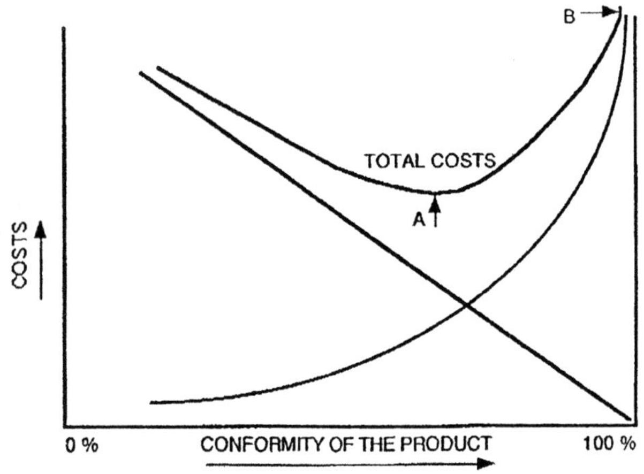

Figure 1.

reporting requirements, I found 29 cases through 1991, but only one had been reported to the FDA.[1] Other evidence of underreporting comes from the reports of errors from New York State published by dr. Linden et al.[2] There is information out there, that is not being used in the way that the FDA intended. So, I suggest that underreporting is happening.

H.I. Hannema (Amsterdam, NL): Mr. Bremer, when one switches from Taylor management system to people oriented quality management what will be the influence on the costs?

H. Bremer: Most of you might be familiar with the graph as shown here in Figure 1.

In order to realize zero defects, the total costs will rise to infinity (B) with the prevention costs (e.g. education and training as well as inspection etc.) also rising enormously. The failure costs, however, will decrease rapidly. If the prevention costs are decreased, the failure costs will increase. It is easy to see that the total costs have a minimum value (A) at a certain level of conformity of the product. This inspection and Taylor oriented graph shows clearly that in order to arrive at a "close to zero defects point" (conformity = 100%) the costs will be skyhigh. For blood banks, this is a serious issue for consideration! It is also easy to understand that implementing a QA system, the costs can be reduced substan-

1. Sazama K, Holland PV. Transfusion-induced graft-versus-host disease. In: Garraty G (ed). Immunobiology of transfusion medicine. Marcel-Dekker publ., New York 1994: 631-56.
2. Linden JV, Paul B, Dressler KP. A report of 104 transfusion errors in New York state. Transfusion 1992;32:601-6.

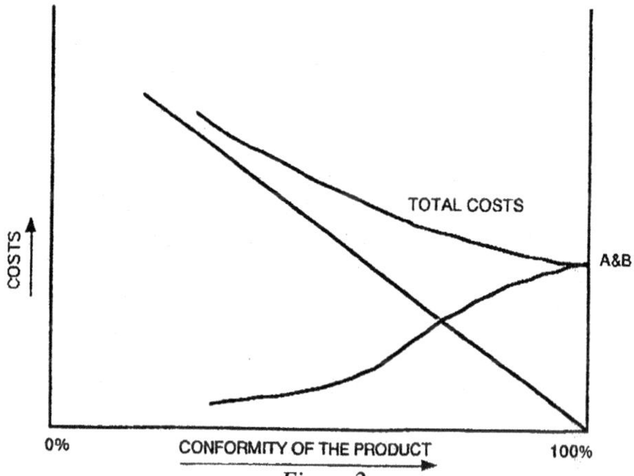

Figure 2.

tially. Implementing market and people oriented TQM in the right way, however, will reduce the costs in a dramatic way as Figure 2 shows.

The prevention costs will not increase as in Figure 1 to infinity, simply because of the fact that the brains of all productive employees are used to improve all processes from top to bottom. It is proven that in organizations where TQM is implemented in the right way, the total costs will show a minimum at zero defects! Close to 100% good products at the lowest possible costs. Here we must be aware that it takes as an average over 10 years to arrive at this point. It should be clear that nobody can quarantee, and will reach zero defects, at a continuous base. Nevertheless, anyone responsible for an organization must realize that he has the choice between the concept as shown in Figures 1 and 2.

T.F. Zuck: The resistance in the United States to cGMP was at the level of the physicians at the hospitals and some of the blood centers. There were papers written about this. Menitove[1] and Polesky[2] wrote editorials about the fact that cGMPs are destroying medical practice. It is making people uninterested in going into medicine: It is not just not a good thing, it is a bad thing. What I am suggesting is that medical organizations should organize in such a way as to retain the medical decision-making of physicians and have a standard of care governing their activities. Blood processing and distribution organizationally should be organized in a totally separate part of the organization based on the good manufacturing practice's rules. Our blood center is set up this way.

1. Menitove JE. The recent emphasis on good manufacturing practices and the pharmaceutical manufacturing approach damages blood banking and transfusion medicine as medical care activities: Con. Transfusion 1993;33:439-42.
2. Polesky HF. Continuous flow. Baxter Deerfield IL 1993;Jan-Feb:4,8.

H.J. Heiniger: Dr. Zuck, would you in the concept of TQM also include the medical clinical part GCP and would that become the overall standard?

T.F. Zuck: Sure, GCP is going to become the medical standard.

H.J. Heiniger: So that the antagonism will disappear?

T.F. Zuck: That is my desire, that is everybody's desire to have physicians co-operate with pharmacists instead of fighting.

E. Vasconcelos (Lisbon, P): Dr. Zuck, do you mean that the blood processing is run by a non-medical staff?

T.F. Zuck: That is absolutely correct. He reports to me, but he is a non-medical person.

E. Vasconcelos: Do you think that we will create a gap between the two departments?

T.F. Zuck: Yes, initially it does somewhat, but it is not posing a problem. Somewhere in the chain of the manufacturing I think you need to get away with the concept that a physician has to run that side of the house. The issue is that the medical issues, that is medical decisions that influence patient care, can be decided by the transfusion medicine specialist, a physician or a physician consultation from the medical advisory board or a medical consultation from one of the physicians on staff.

E. Vasconcelos: Do you think that an other approach would be to train medical doctors in manufacturing or put the manufacturing in their training curriculum.

T.F. Zuck: But that is what doctors do not want to do. You cannot force people to accept cGMP. It has to be a cultural change. But I do not think you could force it on physicians. I think you have to organize around it.

K. Sazama: There is some value in thinking about people who are interested in it. Certainly dr. Zuck is a classic example of a physician who understands good manufacturing practices. He stands right there with that right credential. But I also agree with him that not every physician adopts, or accepts or is even interested in having those kinds of responsibilities. If I can paraphrase what I think he would say: It really depends on matching the person with the interest and the ability with the activity that needs to be done. That person could be a physician or it could be a non-physician. But one needs to be attentive to the fact that, if it is a physician, then the physician has to understand and comply with these requirements. That understanding and compliance is not found necessarily in every transfusion medicine practioner in the United States.

E. Vasconcelos: Dr. Smit Sibinga, can you give me any idea of the GMP. How are the GMP applied in Europe. I mean in every country are they compulsive or just advisable.

C.Th. Smit Sibinga: I cannot really speak for every individual country in Europe. Neither for the Community nor for the Council, nor for a larger Europe, but I know that increasingly, in the Economical Community group of countries, there is implementation ongoing of GMP in the medical field and specifically in the blood banking community. One country is a little further down the road than the other country. In the UK and Scotland one is for instance very active in this respect. The French are active because of their disaster. In the Netherlands this concept has been instituted and in close cooperation with the Health Inspectorate and the Council of Blood Transfusion, the Federation of Red Cross Blood Banks and the Netherlands Society of Blood Transfusion, we try to implement this in more detail in our centers. So, in various countries there is activity on, but it is definitely not yet fully in place nor optimally functioning.

II. Legislative and Regulatory Aspects

EUROPEAN COMMUNITY ACTION ON GOOD MANUFACTURING PRACTICE: CONSUMER PROTECTION AND PRODUCT LIABILITY

L. Gormley

Introduction

The European Community's rules on Good Manufacturing Practice (GMP) are set out in Commission Directive 91/356 [1] which lays down the principles and guidelines of good manufacturing practice for medicinal products for human use. As human blood and human blood products are "substances" within the meaning of Article 1(2) of Directive 65/65 (as amended) [2] they are medicinal products within the meaning of that Directive. Their manufacture or importation into the Community from third countries is thus subject to the holding of an authorization. As an authorization is required under Article 16 of Directive 75/319 [3] the principles and guidelines of GMP apply to medical products derived from human blood or human plasma; such medicinal products include in particular albumin, coagulating factors and immunoglobulins of human origin. However, whole blood, plasma and blood cells of human origin are not covered by Directive 89/381 [4] which enlarged the scope of earlier legislation. Such items are not considered medicinal products within the scope of Community legislation.

The classification of derivatives of human blood or human plasma as products had been the subject of particular controversy. Thus in the "European Agreement on the exchange of therapeutic substances of human origin" (concluded under the aegis of the Council of Europe) [5] the term "product" is avoided by the use of the phrase "therapeutic substances of human origin" to refer to human blood and its derivatives. The Community acceded to that Agreement in 1986 [6]. Despite the controversy over terminology, from the point of view of Directive 85/374 [7] on product liability whole blood, plasma and blood cells of human origin are moveables and thus fall within the rather broad concept of a product enshrined in that directive.

It should not be thought, however, that the Community perceives human blood or human plasma as a product like any other product. Thus the particular interest in the promotion of the humanitarian gesture which the giving of blood represents is expressly acknowledged in Community legislation. Member States are under an obligation under Article 3(4) of Directive 89/381 to take the necessary measures to promote Community self-sufficiency in human blood or human plasma – an obligation incidentally which is leading tot GATT problems with the United States. To this end the Member States are obliged to encourage the voluntary unpaid donation of blood and plasma and to take the necessary measures to develop the production and use of products derived from human blood or human plasma coming from such voluntary unpaid donations. The measures taken have to be notified to the Commission.

The Community definition of GMP

Good manufacturing practice is defined as "the part of Quality Assurance (QA) which ensures that products are consistently produced in the quality standards appropriate to their intended use". In interpreting the principles and guidelines of GMP, manufacturers and national officials are to have regard to the Guide to GMP issued by the Commission and the annexes to that guide [8]. In relation to blood products a new annex to the guide was adopted in December 1992 and came into force in July 1993 [9]. The Member States are obliged to ensure compliance with the principles and guidelines of GMP by means of the repeated inspections by which compliance with the legal requirements relating to medicinal products is ensured. The onus is on the manufacturer to ensure that manufacturing operations are carried out in accordance with GMP and with the manufacturing authorization. As far as medicinal products imported from third countries, the importer is obliged to ensure that they have been manufactured by manufacturers authorized and conforming to GMP standards at least equivalent to those laid down by the European Community. Where appropriate arrangements have been made between the Community with the exporting country to ensure that manufacturers there apply GMP standards equivalent to those of the Community, and that the necessary qualitative, quantitative and other controls have been carried out in the exporting country, the qualified person responsible controlling imported products may be relieved of responsibility for carrying out the controls which would otherwise be required.

Manufacturer's responsibilities

Manufacturers are responsible for ensuring that all manufacturing operations subject to a marketing authorization are carried out in accordance with the information given in the application for the authorization which has been granted by the competent authorities. They must furthermore review regularly their manufacturing methods in the light of scientific and technical progress and any necessary applications for modifications to the marketing authorization dossier must be submitted to the competent authorities. An effective pharmaceutical QA system must be instituted, involving the active participation of the management and personnel of the different services involved. Manufacturers are obliged to have a sufficient number of competent and appropriately qualified personnel at their disposal in sufficient numbers to achieve the objective of pharmaceutical QA. The duties of managerial and supervisory staff, including the qualified persons responsible for implementing and operating GMP have to be defined in job descriptions; the hierarchical relationships must be laid down in an organization chart; both job descriptions and organization charts have to be approved in accordance with the manufacturer's internal procedures and the staff concerned have to be given sufficient authority to discharge their authority correctly. The importance not merely of correct procedures but of motivation and training of personnel is recognized by the requirement of initial and continuing training in QA and GMP. The importance of the personnel is further recognized by the requirement that appropriate hygiene programs be established and observed, including procedures relating to health hygiene and clothing of the personnel.

GMP requires that the location, design, construction, adaptation and maintenance of premises and manufacturing equipment suit the intended operations and that the lay out, design and operation must aim to minimize the risk of errors and permit effective cleaning and maintenance in order to avoid contamination, cross-contamination and, in general, any adverse effect on the quality of the product. In relation to manufacturing operations critical for the quality of products, the premises and equipment intended to be used must be subjected to appropriate qualification. With a view to tracing the history of products the adequacy and accuracy of documentation, including specific batch documentation is particularly important. Thus Directive 91/536 requires that batch documentation be kept *either* for at least a year after the expiry date of the batches to which it relates, *or* at least five years after the certification in accordance with Article 22 of Directive 75/319, whichever period is the longer. Data stored by electronic, photographic or other data processing systems must be appropriately stored during the anticipated storage period, it must be readily available in legible form and protected, for example by duplication or back-up and transfer, against loss or damage.

The different production operations must be carried out according to pre-established instructions and procedures and in accordance with GMP. Manufacturers are obliged to ensure that there are adequate and sufficient resources for the in-process controls. Clearly, it is no good having all the formal structures in the world if there are not enough financial, material and personnel resources to ensure that in-process controls can operate effectively. Appropriate technical and/or organizational measures must be taken to avoid cross-contamination and mix-ups, and any new manufacture or important modification of a manufacturing process must be validated with critical phases being regularly revalidated.

Manufacturers must establish and maintain a QA department which must be independent of the other departments and under the authority of a person having the required qualifications. That department must have at its disposal one or more appropriately staffed and equipped quality control laboratories to carry out the necessary examination and testing of starting materials, packaging materials and intermediate and finished products testing. Outside laboratories may be authorized to conduct the quality control operations under the specific conditions for contracting work out. In particular, the outside laboratories must have clearly defined responsibilities and must observe GMP. Quality control assessment during the final control of finished products before their release for sale or distribution takes into account, in addition to analytical results, essential information such as the production conditions; the results of in-process controls; the examination of the manufacturing documents, and the conformity of the products to their specifications (including the final finished pack). Batch samples must be retained for at least a year after the expiry date and, unless the particular Member State of manufacture requires a longer period, samples of starting materials used (other than solvents, gases and water) have to be retained for at least two years after the release of the products, although if their stability is shorter than two years they may be disposed of at the end of their period of stability. All the samples have to be kept at the disposal of the competent authorities. However, other sampling and retaining conditions may be agreed with the competent authorities in cases of certain products manufactured individually or in small quantities or when storage could raise special problems.

Manufacturers must implement a system for recording and reviewing complaints, together with an effective and prompt product recall system for medicinal products in the distribution network. Complaints concerning defects must be recorded and investigated by the manufacturer, who must inform the competent authority of any defect that could result in a recall or abnormal restriction on the supply of the product concerned. In so far as possible the countries of destination must also be indicated. The person responsible for marketing a medicinal product must inform the Member States concerned of suspension of marketing or withdrawal of a product from the market, together with the reasons for such action if they concern the efficacy of the product or the protection of public health. Both the Commission and the Committee for Proprietary Medicinal Products have to be informed in such cases by the Member States, who must also ensure that suspension or withdrawal of a product in these circumstances is brought to the attention of the WHO if it could affect the protection of public health in third countries. The Commission has the additional responsibility of publishing annually a list of the medicinal products which are prohibited in the Community.

Finally, Directive 91/356 obliges manufacturers to conduct repeated self-inspection systems as part of their QA system in order to monitor the implementation and respect of GMP and to propose any necessary corrective measures. Records of such self-inspections and any subsequent corrective action must be kept.

Product liability

As far as Directive 85/374 on product liability, there are one or two features of that regime which deserve specific attention here. First, the system is based on the concept of no-fault liability. Secondly the directive embraces a very broad concept of a producer, namely the manufacturer of a finished product, the producer of any raw material, the manufacturer of any component part, and any person who, by putting his name, trade mark or other distinguishing feature on the product presents himself as its producer; the definition of a producer also extends to include an importer into the Community of a product for sale, hire, leasing or any form of distribution in the course of his business. Where the producer of the product cannot be identified, each supplier of the product is treated as its producer, and is thus liable for damage caused by defects, unless he within a reasonable time informs the injured person of the identity of the producer or of the person who supplied him with the product. The same applies in respect of a product imported from a third country if the product does not indicate the identity of the importer, even if it does indicate the name of the producer.

The concrete issue which is of concern is the extent of the liability of a blood transfusion service for the supply of blood. Given that the product liability directive treats blood as a product; the answer is, therefore, that where the injured person can prove the causal relationship between the defect and the damage, liability will most likely be with the supplier. Whilst some might think of a blood donor as a producer of a raw material, it is inconceivable that an individual blood donor can be fixed with liability in the sense of the directive. Blood in a transfusion is almost certainly going to come from more than one donor and it may not always be possible to identify which donor is the originator of the blood. Such liability as a donor may incur is more likely to be in the criminal field (if it can be shown that the donor knowingly gave infected blood) or under any special liability system already existing on July 30, 1985 when the product liability directive was notified to the Member States. Given that all blood taken is now systematically tested and given the controls through the application of GMP in the manufacture of products derived from human blood or human plasma, the question is hopefully merely academic, but it appears that the transfusion service is liable under the Directive, save to the extent to which its activities are covered by Article 7(c). This excludes liability if the producer proves that the product was neither manufactured by him for sale nor any form of distribution for economic purpose nor manufactured or distributed by him in the course of his business. In so far as blood derivatives are concerned, which are the subject of commercial operations, the activities of blood banks – even of the Red Cross – are covered by the directive. Even if it argued, on the basis of the European Agreement on the Exchange of Therapeutic Substances of Human Origin, that the restriction to charging "only those costs involved in the collection, processing and carriage" of such substances means that their production does not constitute an "economic purpose" it appears difficult to argue that they are not produced in the course of a business. The mere fact that an operation is not carried on for profit does not automatically mean that it has no economic purpose. At least, then, in so far as commercial operations are concerned, it seems that liability under the product liability directive is inevitable. As yet, however, there is no case-law of the Court of Justice of the European Communities on the point. A point which should not be overlooked, though, is the possible availability (depending on whether the Member State concerned has used the possibility provided for in Article 15(1)(b) of the directive) of the "state of the art" defence. The Member States may or may not provide for liability irrespective of proof by the producer "that the state of scientific and technical knowledge at the time when he put the product into circulation was not such as to enable the existence of a defect to be discovered".

Conclusions

The Community's rules on GMP provide a framework within which the legitimate health concerns of Community citizens can be guaranteed as far as possible. Proper compliance with those provisions affords an incentive to free movement of blood and blood derivatives within the Community, facilitating the expression of solidarity with areas of the Community which have a considerable shortage of blood donations [10]. In so far at least as the clearly commercial activities of voluntary blood banks are concerned, liability under the product liability directive seems certain. In so far as their other activities are concerned, whilst there is no authority on the point, it would be too unwise to conclude at this stage that there is absolutely no possibility of liability accruing for non-commercial activities. Whilst non-liability may undoubtedly be convenient for some, it is not a horse on which too much money should be bet.

References

1. O.J. 1991;L193/30.
2. O.J. 1965;22/369, most recently amended by Directive 93/39 (O.J. 1993;L214/22.
3. O.J. 1975;L147/13.
4. Art. 1(2), O.J. 1989;L181/44.
5. The text of the Agreement is conveniently reproduced in O.J. 1986;L207/2. An additional protocol to the Agreement made it possible for the Community to become a contracting party (see note 6. *infra*).
6. By Decision 86/346 (O.J. 1986;L207/1). See also the European Agreement on the Exchange of Blood-grouping Reagents, accepted by the Community by Dec. 86/347 (O.J. 1986;L207/30). the text of this latter Agreement is reproduced in O.J. 1986;L207/31.
7. O.J. 1985;L210/29.
8. The latest issue of the Guide is dated January 1992, forming Volume IV of the Rules governing Medicinal Products in the European Community. Volume I has been revised to November 1993 and applies from January 1, 1995. See also Volume III addendum 2 (May 1992), in particular the guidelines on Medicinal Products derived from blood and plasma (dating from December 1991) and on Validation of virus removal and inactivation procedures (dating from May 1991). Note that the general chapters of the Guide apply to products derived from human blood or plasma, unless otherwise stated. Some of the other annexes may also apply, e.g. those on the manufacture of sterile medicinal products, the use of ionizing radiation in the manufacture of medicinal products, and the annex on biological medicinal products.
9. Manufacture of products derived from human blood or human plasma (Commission document III/3232/92-EN of December 22, 1992). Because several provisions of this annex apply equally to plasma and products derived therefrom, to cellular components and to whole blood, an additional paragraph relating to the latter two only has been included in this annex for the convenience of those competent authorities wishing to control those components (points 27-29). Those components are, however, outside the scope of present Community pharmaceutical legislation (as was noted at the begin-

ning of this paper). No special provisions covering the manufacture of medicinal products derived from placental blood are included in this annex, although all the relevant provisions of the guide to GMP apply to their manufacture.

10. See, generally, Sauer (1992) Le donneur de sang bénévole no. 24.

REGULATORY SYSTEMS AND MECHANISMS

H.I. Hannema

Introduction

You have travelled to Groningen. It is almost impossible to come here without noticing that you are in the European Community (EC). If you came by car or train you must have noticed that there was no border-control, neither in Germany nor in Belgium. If you came by plane you have seen that there are special gates for holders of EC passports and these gates are usually fast and easy. Within a few months there will be no longer controls at the airports for trips between nine of the twelve EC-countries. The EC affects many aspects of our daily life. But the EC also affects our professional life.

The EC was founded in 1958 with the purpose of creating a common market for all participating countries. These countries are usually called Member States. The common market was defined as the free circulation of goods, the free circulation of persons and the free circulation of services. The means to achieve this was the removal of all existing barriers through harmonization of national legislation. Another important principle is that EC legislation prevails over national legislation. The EC legislation is contained in so called directives. In the first twenty years of its existence the development of the common market was relatively slow. In the eighties the EC got a new impetus when the creation of a single market in 1992 was announced. A so-called whitebook was made which listed all products which could not yet circulate freely. Blood products were one group of those products. As a consequence a special EC directive for blood products was made. But the eighties were also the years when AIDS and HIV were discovered. All Member States were involved and blood products became a hot item for politicians. As you may well know the problem was biggest in France. Blood bankers and even two former ministers and a former prime minister were taken to court. This year we all read in the newspapers that France will change its constitution in order to facilitate the prosecution of ministers.

The result of these developments was that the directive on blood products could not resolve all problems [1]. This is demonstrated most clearly by the fact that several groups of blood products were excluded from the harmonization regime. These products are whole blood, plasma, cellular products and placental products. Whole blood and cellular products were left out because no Member

State required registration. Furthermore the need for free circulation seemed limited, because of their relatively short stability. Plasma was left out as this was considered to be an intermediate, which is already more difficult to understand, because many problems came from infected plasma, especially plasma which had been imported into the Community. Placental products were left out for a completely different reason. It was not possible to reach an agreement between the Member States. Some states allowed placental products, because they thought that the virus inactivation method was sufficient. Other states wanted the double check which is being used with other products: testing of the donor and virus inactivation. The harmonization of national legislation was achieved by requiring that the general legal regime for medicinal products should apply to blood products. This regime includes licensing, registration, labelling and Good Manufacturing Practice (GMP). Secondly some special requirements for blood products were introduced:

- Uniform declaration of contents;
- Virus inactivation or removal procedures;
- Promotion of self-sufficiency;
- Traceability;
- State control of bulk products and/or finished products;
- EC registration of products.

Three of these special requirements need some comment. The statement about the promotion of self-sufficiency has not had any effect, as far as I can see. The reason is that no concrete measures were imposed on Member States. Self-sufficiency is of course self-sufficiency of the EC. The state control of bulk products and/or finished products has been interpreted in different ways in the various Member States. Some states require that every batch of every product be tested, other states require testing only for some products. But all states respect each others tests. The introduction of an EC registration in stead of national registration is new for these products, but the system of an EC registration had already been introduced for other products, like biotechnological products.

This short introduction to EC harmonization may have given an impression of what the effect of the single market is on blood products. Much work has been done, but it is very clear that not all problems have been solved yet.

Annex for blood products of the EC GMP guide [2]

When the decision was taken that blood products should be seen as medicinal products for legal purposes, it also included the decision that the GMP guide should apply. But the EC authorities were aware of the special character of the products and they suggested that some special provisions for blood products should be mentioned in the annex on biotechnological products. Several Member States found that the two subjects did not have enough in common. At a meeting in Copenhagen, it was decided that a special annex for blood products should be written.

The EC authorities then invited the Member States to send their experts on blood products to Brussels. Some of the experts had done some home-work and made a list of subjects to be covered in the annex. A rapporteur was elected having the task of making the draft of the annex and defending the draft for the EC authorities and of making the necessary modifications. The final responsibility for the text remains, however, with the European Commission. In other words the rapporteur works on behalf of the Commission and reports to the Commission.

First two fundamental decisions were taken. The first decision was that the annex should be drafted in accordance with the leading principle of the GMP guide, that general requirements should be formulated and that details, especially quantitative requirements, should not be introduced into the text. This decision proved to be difficult to maintain. Those countries which had big problems with AIDS in the blood supply, were not in favour of this decision. It is my impression that this resistance was mainly politically motivated. The text of the annex shows the results of the struggle, but the general idea has been maintained.

The second decision was to include cellular products. This was a very remarkable step. Here the technicians demonstrated the wish to harmonize the requirements, without a previous legal base to do so. The EC authorities showed some doubt about the legality of the decision, but is was indeed remarkable that all experts who were involved in the drafting of the text, had no problem in reaching an agreement on the text.

No agreement could be reached on placental products. In the Community there is only one industry which produces products derived from human placentas. Some Member States do not allow these products on the market. It is my impression that this could be overcome if an agreement could be reached on two technical subjects, the permission of the donor to use the placenta and the testing of the donor. However, there was no way out. Therefore the annex does not apply to placental products.

Of the topics in the annex the most important ones are to be discussed. The first issue is that the principles of quality management from the chapter 1 of the GMP guide apply. This is not stated in the annex. The general chapters 1 to 9 always apply to all annexes. The main issues of quality management are the following:

- Quality Assurance (QA) covers all aspects;
- There is a head of production and a head of quality control;
- They are normally full-time employed, except in collection centers;
- They are independent of each other;
- They have some shared or jointly exercised responsibilities related to quality.

This concept is rather new in the world of blood transfusion. Often no clear distinction was made between in-process controls and quality controls. In some cases the personnel has rotating jobs between the various departments. Approval and release of finished products has often been seen as a routine job, best done by a computer. The GMP idea of quality management will change the traditional quality views of blood banks.

A second important idea is found in paragraph 4 of the annex. The full text of paragraph 4 is: "Results of the controls carried out on the accepted donors should be part of the quality documentation of the collecting center and should be available to the manufacturer".

The first topic addressed in this paragraph is the implicit statement that the donor is the starting material. This is the only place in the GMP guide where such a (clear) definition of the starting material has been made.

The second topic addressed in this paragraph is the matter of confidentiality. The importance of safe donations is so big, that it must be guaranteed. It must be realized that the EC imports 35-50 per cent of its plasma and that this plasma is often from paid donors. The relevant aspects of safe donations are:

- Donors using more names or false names;
- Too frequent donations;
- Donations at more collecting centers;
- Reliability of the donor interview.

In order to gain the confidence of the donor it is important to keep in touch and provide information. To guarantee the safety of the donation the donor should agree with the restricted confidentiality of the results. Obviously it is not necessary to reveal the name of the donor.

A third topic addressed in this paragraph is the implicit statement that the manufacturer nor the authorities have to be informed of results of rejected donors. In terms of patient rights this means that infectious diseases like AIDS do not have to be reported, especially not to the authorities. There is already enough discrimination of people with AIDS.

Also of importance is paragraph 3, which states that dedicated facilities should be used. This is a recognition of the fact that collection and processing of blood products is a highly specialized technique and that it is so vulnerable that dedicated facilities are warranted. There are, however, two exceptions:

- Blood collection may be done on a mobile team basis;
- Packaging operations where the contents are in a closed container can be executed under normal precautions. Obviously the collection of blood and the processing in closed systems are not considered to be packaging operations.

A fourth idea which is mentioned in the annex is the statement in paragraph 13. This paragraph states that products and intermediates must be tested and found non-reactive for some micro-organisms before issuing or fractionation. This paragraph is in my view superfluous because it is already completely covered by the general chapters of the GMP guide. However, this paragraph is of relevance because it was introduced under the pressure of countries with major AIDS problems. To complete the picture, this was also the case of paragraphs 20 to 25, which are quotations from the registration guidelines (notes for guidance in the language used by the EC).

There is one more issue. It is expected that the EC will be expanded to more Member States, like Austria, Finland, Malta, Sweden and maybe some more countries. Already now an agreement has been reached with countries adhering to the Pharmaceutical Inspection Convention (PIC). They have accepted the EC GMP guide and are also expected to accept new additions and modifications. With exception of the EC Member States these countries are now Australia, Austria, Czech Republic, Finland, Hungary, Iceland, Norway, Slovakia, Sweden and Switzerland (Figure 1).

It is interesting to compare how many inhabitants the various countries do have. The EC Member States do have 345 million inhabitants. The PIC countries do have an additional number of inhabitants of 75 million. The GMP annex on blood products is therefore applicable to a population size of 420 million. If this number is compared to the USA with 242 million inhabitants and Japan with 122 million inhabitants, the importance of the EC GMP guide becomes very clear.

New Dutch legislation for clinical use [3]

The last theme to discuss is a recent national legislation in the Netherlands. The efforts by the EC to obtain harmonization leads to changes in national legislation in many Member States. This happened also in the Netherlands. The existing law will be changed again in the Parliament, but already detailed requirements put down in decrees have been established. A new and recent decree has a chapter on the handling of blood and blood products in hospitals. So far no experience has been obtained with this chapter because it is extremely recent. Assuming that many do work in hospitals, it might therefore be of interest to know what this new chapter is meant to accomplish.

The most important issue is that hospitals should seek for economical and efficient use of blood and blood products. Two elements of this text, i.e. the words hospital and economical are of particular interest.

The text begins with the word hospitals. This means that this is a task for the management of the hospital. The clinicians are not addressed, but it is of course impossible for the hospitals to carry out the obligation without addressing the physician. There are a few management tools already in use in Dutch hospitals. One of them is that only one unit of a blood product at a time is being distributed to the ward. For operating rooms there are usually standard quantities for the various operations. For emergencies it will usually not be possible to establish standard quantities.

The second element is the economical use of blood and blood products. This matter is even more difficult to address. The idea of the legislator is clear. The donor has given his blood and it is the obligation of all involved that the blood is used for the purposes it was given for. It should not remain in stock until it is outdated, but neither should it be given when it is not needed. This addresses the matter of the indication. It will therefore be necessary to establish indications for the blood products and, not less important, see that these are adhered to. This re-

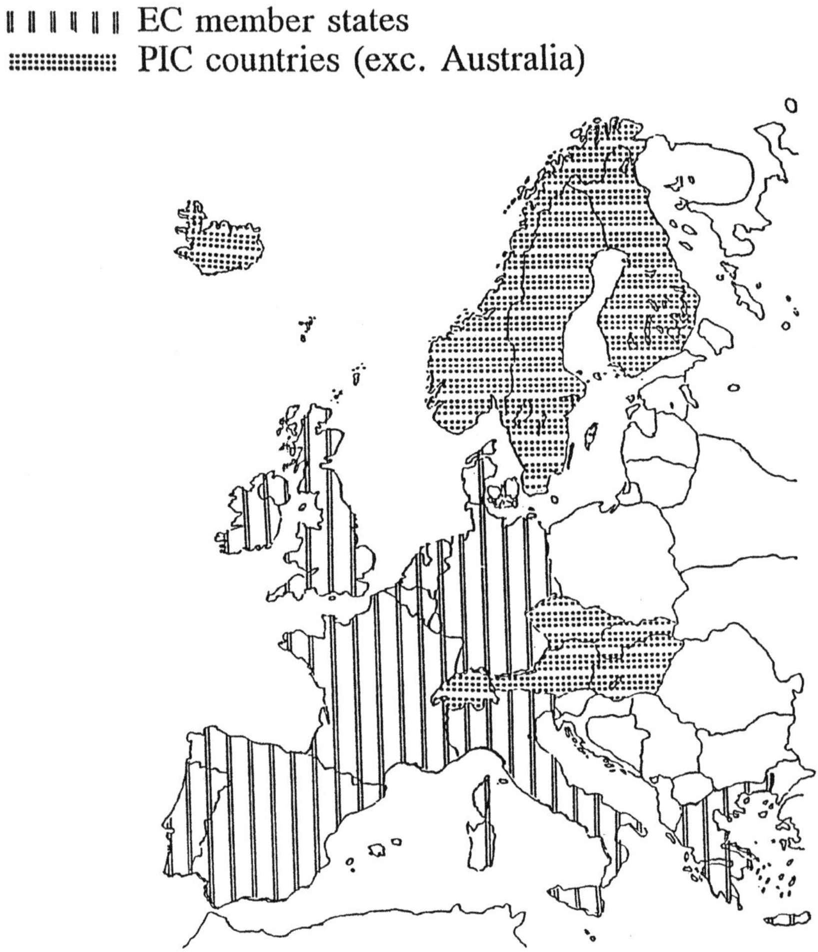
EC member states
PIC countries (exc. Australia)

quires that the hospital must have a system to monitor the adherence to the established indications. One way of achieving this is to discuss the use in a blood transfusion committee within the hospital. To put this on the agenda of the committee the distributor, usually the clinical chemist or the pharmacist, should bring the case forward. These discussions will not be easy, but we do have a good example in this country with drugs. To minimize the cost of the drugs in this country the hospital pharmacist has already a long experience of how to influence the prescription behaviour of the clinician. So far this has not been the case with the use of blood products, but this new legislation could stimulate. Much will also depend on how the new legislation will be implemented. Time and patience will certainly be important factors.

The other elements of the new Dutch requirements in the hospital paragraph are much less far reaching. They include the prescription, the traceability, the labelling and the equipment.

The internal distribution of blood products on a medical prescription only seems rather classic. However, in practice many variations are seen. Nurses write the prescription or sometimes the prescription is given by telephone only. A document signed by the clinician is necessary for the record and to protect the nurses against a responsibility which they can not carry.

The requirement of traceability in the hospital is a consequence of the EC guidelines. It must be possible to trace a donation to a patient and vice versa. It should not be necessary to carry out a long search in hospital archives to find the information. This will imply that the distributor in the hospital, the clinical chemist or the pharmacist keeps a record of all distributions to all patients.

The requirement of labelling is obvious and needs no comment. The text on the label put onto the product in the hospital should include the patients name and where applicable day and hour of issuing.

Equipment used for handling of blood products, thawing baths, refrigerators etc. should comply with GMP requirements for equipment.

The last issue is the cross matching and other screening methods of blood products. This issue is not addressed in the new regulations because the legal basis is lacking. However, this does not mean that the subject is less important.

References

1. Directive 89/381/EEC.
2. Anonymous. The rules governing medicinal products in the EC. 1993;vol IV.
3. Staatscourant 1993;12 Oct:195.

GOOD MANUFACTURING PRACTICE AND BLOOD DERIVATIVES: REQUIREMENTS AND MECHANISMS FOR PRODUCT LICENSING

J.M. Noel, Y. Dumas

One of the aims of public health systems consists in guaranteeing access to effective, safe and high quality products for all people suffering from illness throughout the world. The achievement (or non-achievement) of this overall quality objective entirely depends on Good Manufacturing Practices (GMP). Moreover, these GMPs themselves form an integral component of the concept of Quality Assurance (QA), within which they are combined with Good Laboratory Practice (GLP) and Good Clinical Practice (GCP). All of these good practice principles define the conditions in which a product must be designed and managed from the time it is conceived to the time of its eventual use. Where GMPs themselves are concerned, these specifically deal with all that embraces production up to and including the eventual time of distribution of each unit manufactured.

GMP as part of the QA system

It is possible to draw a chart of the relationships between the various concepts (Figure 1). This diagrammatical representation is completely artificial in that each field interrelates with each of the two others at one level or another. It nevertheless enables us to grasp clearly the fields of activity: Firstly, that covered by the whole concept and, secondly, that covered by each internal field. QA manages quality as a whole, while GMP manages quality with respect to the

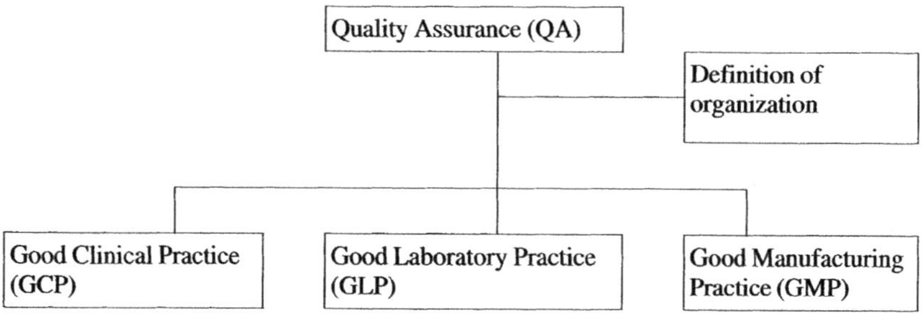

Figure 1.

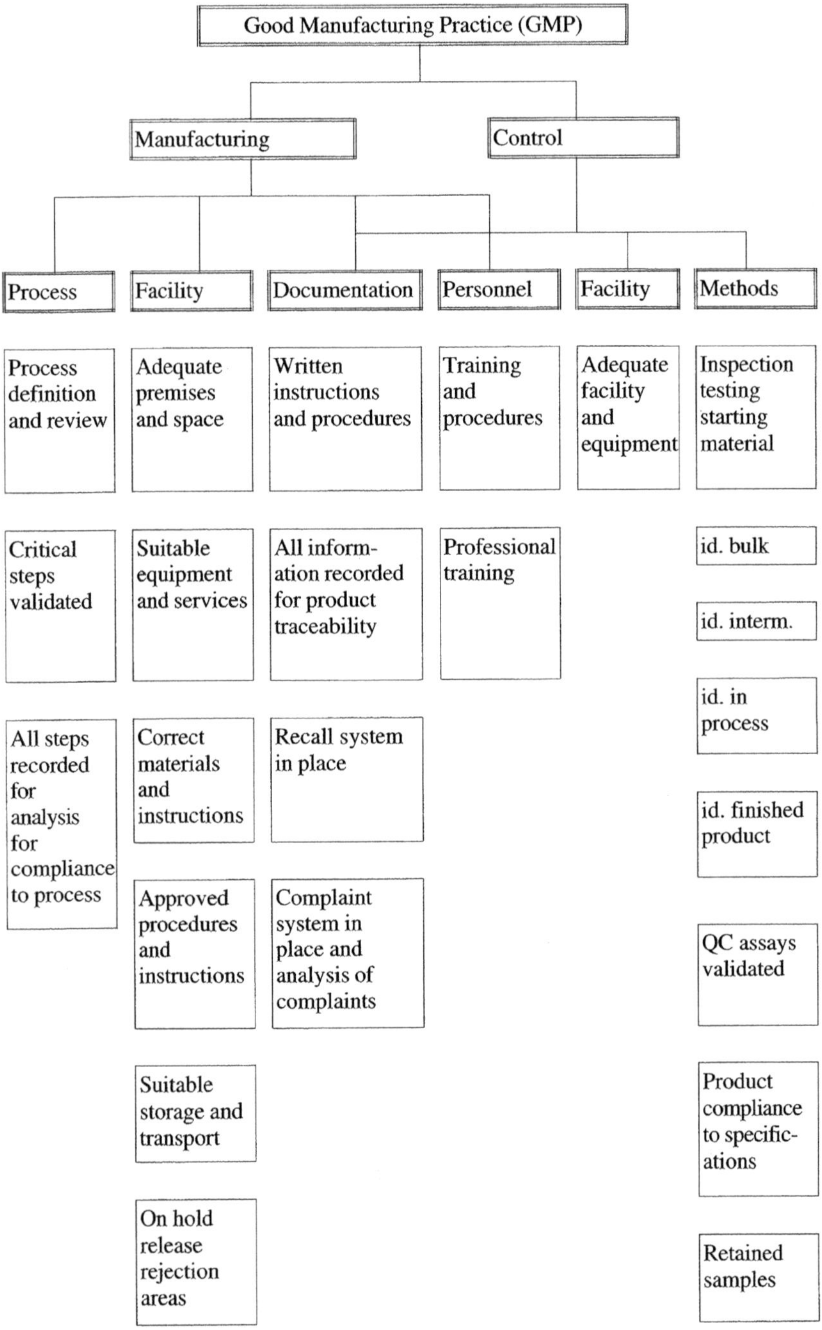
Good Manufacturing Practice (GMP)
Manufacturing
Control
Process
Facility
Documentation
Personnel
Facility
Methods
Process definition and review
Critical steps validated
All steps recorded for analysis for compliance to process
Adequate premises and space
Suitable equipment and services
Correct materials and instructions
Approved procedures and instructions
Suitable storage and transport
On hold release rejection areas
Written instructions and procedures
All inform-ation recorded for product traceability
Recall system in place
Complaint system in place and analysis of complaints
Training and procedures
Professional training
Adequate facility and equipment
Inspection testing starting material
id. bulk
id. interm.
id. in process
id. finished product
QC assays validated
Product compliance to specific-ations
Retained samples

Figure 2.

manufacturing of products. Although it may be unusual, it seems necessary to specify that the overall concept as well as each subconcept, requires clear and precise definition of organization and of responsibilities (who does what in which structure), implying definitions with respect to positions held and to matters requiring decisions.

GMP as an overall concept and definition of the fields affected by product licensing

In that GMPs directive affect the field of "production" for any product, they basically include manufacturing and quality control (Figure 2). Though it is difficult to be comprehensive in such a table summarizing what GMPs are, such a presentation nevertheless enables us to define the basic fields covered by individual GMPs.

GMP: The supplier and the manufacturer

In that GMPs constitute an integral component of the QA program, they must ensure complete traceability of all information associated with all source products used in the production of a finished product or associated with all action carried out during the course of manufacturing a finished product. The final quality of the finished product depends both on guarantees of the quality of each raw material and on the overall quality of the production and finished product testing parameters. It is in the context of such a definition that it is necessary to analyze the constraints applicable to suppliers and manufacturers. Such description enables the requirements and mechanisms necessary in order to achieve "product licensing" to be better understood. As the overall context of GMPs demonstrates, a distinction must be applied between the supplier and the manufacturer. Where blood derivatives are concerned, one can assume the following division (Figure 3).

Blood and plasma	=	Transfusion services and blood banks	=	SUPPLIERS
Fractionation	=	Fractionation centers	=	MANUFACTURERS

Figure 3.

The supplier

The publication of guidelines for QA in blood establishments is required for two main reasons:

1. To make sure that human blood collected and subsequently used for fractionation is treated in standardized conditions resulting in desirable quality and thus enabling quality blood derivatives to be obtained.
2. To comply with the general "Rules governing medicinal products in the EC".

– *The general rules imposed upon the supplier*

Generally, the rules applicable both in the EC and in the USA will refer to:

- Personnel training, education and evaluation;
- Management of all relevant information;
- Equipment;
- Validation;
- Error and accident reports;
- Complaints and adverse event reports.

They will reiterate the notion of QA function, the requirement for definition of the supplier's organization and of the responsibilities of the latter. Matters relating to the size of the supplier's departments are not, generally speaking, matters constituting a part of GMPs. In the same way, matters relating to efficiency and economic feasibility of the supplier's activity do not form a part of them. All these internal regulations must be laid down in writing and known throughout the organization. Considering the experience obtained in other fields, particularly in that of the pharmaceutical industry, one can assume that each supplier will not only have to comply with these regulations, but also obtain a periodically reviewed legal authorization to operate. Considering the extreme sensitivity of this subject within the EC, considering the legal differences between the countries and the still obvious differences between the histories of the EC Member States, one can assume that a system will gradually be put in place

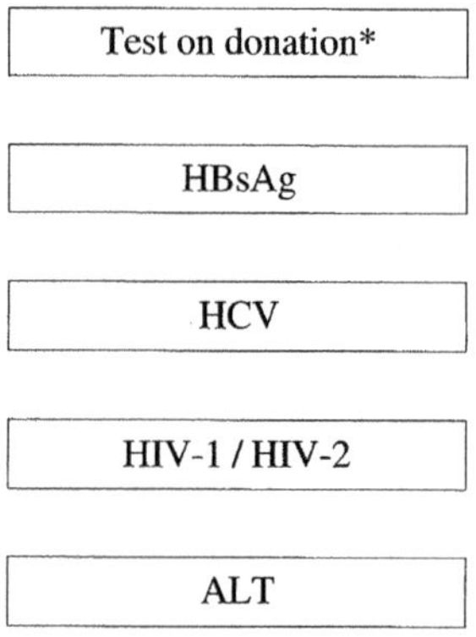

* EC Note for guidance III/3010/93-EN, May, 1993.

Figure 4.

in the context of a very general European guideline implying mutual recognition of national certifications. Each manufacturer will be required to make sure that each supplier is properly certified. In some EC countries, supply of a copy of the certificate will be necessary.

– *Specific rules imposed on the human blood/plasma supplier*

As the main function of the supplier consists in collecting and/or separating plasma, each supplier will have a certain specific number of obligations to fulfil in the context of traceability of information. He will be required to supply the manufacturer with evidence that each blood donation has been tested in accordance with the European requirements (Figure 4). Constant availability of this information, along with certification, forms the fundamental basis of the supplier's undertakings with respect to the manufacturer. All data relevant to testing of donations must be held in records by the supplier for at least one year after the finished product's expiration date. They are the indispensable guarantee of the quality of the raw mateirals required for the manufacture of blood derivatives.

The manufacturer

The manufacturer's role by definition consists in making sure that:

1. The raw materials which he procures comply with the specifications stipulated by the EC.
2. The manufacturing process is correctly validated and enables a finished product of constant and reproducible quality to be obtained.
3. The finished manufactured product complies with the specifications stipulated by the EC.
4. All information generated in the course of the product's production and while it is being used is suitably analyzed and that the corrective action is taken in timely manner where desirable corrections are applicable.

– *General rules imposed on the manufacturer*

These rules derive directly from the GMPs described in the "Rules governing medicinal products in the European Community". Generally, they relate to:

Where production is concerned:

- Definition of the production premises and designation of their uses;
- Description of equipment and resources implemented;
- Description and definition of equipment and labelling;
- Definition of organization and responsibilities;
- The requirement for written operational, dated and approved procedures;
- Process validation;
- Definition of storage and carriage facilities for products;
- Definition of release/hold and rejection notifications. Where inspection is concerned:
- Definition of premises and equipment;
- The requirement for written, dated and approved inspection procedures both for raw materials (if methods are not EP methods) and for intermediate products, in-process inspections as well as finished product inspections;

- Methods validation;
- Analysis of information generated and approval of all action or decisions taken or made with respect to written procedures.

Certain actions are common to both procution and inspection:
- Writing, dating and signing of procedures;
- Analysis and storage of information generated both in the course of production and inspection, and during the commercialization phase;
- Personnel training.

Moreover, a recall, analysis and complaints processing system must be implemented. Complaints must be processed in a documented manner. Some Member States have analytical systems, termed "imputation" systems, which carry out analysis of secondary clinical effects. The matter of the size of fractionation centers does not constitute an integral part of GMPs, and neither do matters of efficiency and economic feasibility. On the basis of the GMPs applied to medicinal products, one can forecast that relatively soon each manufacturer shall be required to obtain an authorization requiring periodical renewal in order to open and operate, on the basis of an assessment of compliance with the GMPs. The historical differences between the Member States do not enable the manner in which this development will take place or its timetable to be precisely predicted. It is probable that it will initially be national, so processes of mutual recognition between Member States are implied.

– *Specific rules imposed on manufacturers of blood derivatives*

These specific rules derive from the general "Rules governing medicinal products in the European Community". They owe their specificity to the very nature of the raw material (blood/plasma = product of biological origin), or to the very nature of the manufacturing processes (fractionation). These can be divided into four groups:
- Fractionation and validation or what guarantees to implement in order to obtain the quality sought after in a product defined by its manufacturing process;
- Manufacture of a purified product, or validation of both a new manufacturing stage and validation of a specific purification step;
- Manufacture from a product potentially contaminated by a virus, or validation of a virus inactivation process;
- Manufacture of a therapeutic product defined by its activity, or how to maintain the biological activity of a product within the desired limits.

Fractionation and validation

Unlike products of synthetic or semi-synthetic origin, for which it is possible to extract intermediate products which are often well defined by physical and/or chemical properties, the fractionation process proceeds in stages. Each product originating from each stage has no precise specification at a physical, chemical or even biological level. Consistency in the quality of each intermediate product therefore depends on strict control of the operating parameters:

- Ethanol/protein concentration;
- Temperatures;
- pH/ionic strength;
- etc.

The operating parameters must therefore be validated and inspection be carried out on each production batch in the context of a defined margin of error. Such validation thus requires precise and regular validation of equipment and measuring resources, plus regular revalidation of the process. This information, according to the guidelines, must form part of the information enabling the product license to be obtained. Any major change in the process must be validated. In order to ensure the success of such an operation, it is always preferable to validate one single change at a time. In these circumstances, validation will be carried out by assessment of the effects of the change implemented on that stage, by assessment of its effects on the subsequent stages, and by its effect on yield and the specification of the finished products.

Manufacturing of a purified product

The development of highly purified product necessitates the use of new techniques requiring a double validation:
- Validation of a new manufacturing stage with its potential repercussions on the physical and biological quality of the finished product;
- Validation of the new stage in terms of both purity, efficacy and product safety.

– *Introduction of a new stage in the production process*

Any change must be validated firstly to ensure that the process can be reproduced and secondly to evaluate the possible effect on the physical and biological properties of the finished product, and thus assess the predictable repercussions for the product quality (specifications and product quality). Such validation cannot be validly carried out until the final process has been definitively assessed on the basis of the effectiveness desired.

– *Validation of the purification process*

In addition to the effectiveness of the process this new manufacturing stage must be validated for the non-contamination of the finished product. Leachables have to be identified and quantified. The most precise process must carefully be set up and followed without new changes being validated. The specifications of the finished product must be carefully documented.

Manufacture and virus inactivation

The very origin of the raw material implies the risk of viral contamination, both by known viruses and by viruses unknown at this time. The inclusion of an inactivation phase requires double validation:

- Validation of a new manufacturing stage with its possible repercussions on the physical and chemical quality of the finished product;
- Validation of the effectiveness of the new stage on the lipid and non-lipid enveloped viruses.

– *Inclusion of a new stage in the production process*

The European guidelines refer to the previous instance. Any change must be validated firstly to ensure that the process can be reproduced and secondly to evaluate the possible effect on the physical and chemical properties of the finished product, and thus assess the predictable repercussions for finished product quality (specification and specific activity). Such validation cannot be validly carried out unless the inactivation process has been definitively assessed and selected on the basis of the effectiveness desired.

– *Validation of virus inactivation*

As a result of GMP constraints, it is not appropriate to carry out such validation on the production premises, as validation of the process requires the plasma to be spiked. It is thus necessary to carry out an assessment in the laboratory under conditions which reproduce the actual process to the best possible extent. The scaling-down parameters need to be clearly specified. Different processes may be used, such as heating to 60°C for 10 hours, freeze-drying, UV irradiation or the addition of chemical substances. In each case the specifications of detailed procedures must be studied and their effectiveness measured on the spiking virus. As a result, it may be necessary to add a virus inactivation phase to an existing process. In order to do so, the performance of the existing process will firstly have to be assessed and compared to the objective sought after. In this respect, the requirements of the guidelines are imprecise, varying from a minimum of 6-8 log reduction up to 12 log reduction. In the same way, selection of the viruses is a matter for discussion, except for HIV-1 and HIV-2. It would actually be more realistic to reduce the risks of a manipulatory accident and carry out this work using model viruses as closely related as possible to the pathogenic viruses, particularly for HCV or HAV.

Manufacture of a defined activity product

Blood derivatives being by definition products specified by the manufacturing process, the nature of the process implies variability in the activity level of the finished product. As a result, these products have been commercialized at their nominal value. Their classification as medicinal products means that the active principle content of the finished product is within the defined acceptable limits approximating the theoretical value. This may obviously be affected by control over the process, its controlled improvement, and the strict implementation of integrated GMP management at all levels. It is naturally the case that the biological origins of the product and the process type would mean that most blood derivatives would have wider-ranging limits than those of chemical products, which are usually set at ca. 5 per cent.

Conclusion

GMP must be regarded not only as rules manufacturers have to comply with, but more importantly as a tool for:

- Empowering people into product R&D and manufacturing;
- Setting up a strong basis for product improvements in understanding as precisely as possible the influence of key factors on the step by step process.

In addition it will be more and more a legal requirement for getting access to market within the European Community.

References

1. Note for guideance, III/3010/93-EN-Draft No. 5, May 1993.
2. The rules governing medicinal products in the European Community. Volume III.
3. The rules governing medicinal products in the European Community. Volume III, Addendum No. 2.
4. The rules governing medicinal products in the European Community. Volume IV.
5. Guideline for quality assurance in blood establishments. Docket nr. 91N-0450-Draft, June 17, 1993.

STANDARDS AND EXTERNAL QUALITY AUDIT SYSTEMS

P.A. Hoppe

Introduction

There are some significant differences between the Unites States of America (USA) and other countries in the standards for blood products, the expectations of regulatory or peer review groups responsible for setting those standards, and the methods for determining whether all facilities comply with the applicable standards. Most workers in all countries would agree, however, that "external audits", (or "inspections" in the blood banker's usual jargon) are a *very* important part of programs aimed at ensuring blood and blood components meet quality standards which have been prospectively agreed upon.

Some peer review groups, such as the American Association of Blood Banks or the Joint Commission on Accreditation of Healthcare Organizations have also had an educational objective, whereas regulatory agencies are primarily inspecting to determine whether the blood bank meets all defined requirements.

The tools for conducting these assessments have varied, but all those of which I am aware have been derived within the same paradigm of periodic on-site observations of practices and records. Reports usually include checklists of important items that the inspector has asked about and a description of problems. It is a time-honoured tradition, and a legal requirement for the Food and Drug Administration (FDA), that the assessment be conducted by someone independent of the facility under review so that there is no interfering "conflict of interest" or other factor which diminishes the likelihood that deficiencies will be discovered and objectively evaluated.

Today we stand at an important juncture in blood bank history and before us lies an unexplored pathway of heightened reliance on Quality Assurance (QA) systems. We expect this new emphasis on QA systems will find better ways to ensure quality products. Many are proposing that concurrently we take a new look at whether there are better ways to evaluate the manufacturers of those products to determine whether there is compliance with all of the standards that have been defined. The AABB inspections and accreditation program, for example, has begun planning for quality systems review.

The US FDA requirements include specific product standards, memoranda conveying Recommendations for Blood Establishments, and current Good

Manufacturing Practices (cGMPs) for producing safe and effective quality products [1]. To some degree, it doesn't even matter what the specific standards are, or how much the standards may vary from one country to the next, because the proposal is generic. Just as the Blood Transfusion Council of the Netherlands Red Cross has succeeded in producing an excellent document, "GMP for blood banks", that can be applied in every setting regardless of the specific procedures in that location, I am optimistic that inspection processes can be similarly addressed [2]. It is time to change the focus of inspection programs from detailed lists of "did or did not" to a broader evaluation of the way in which the facility has planned for, implemented, managed and monitored the QA programs. If carefully defined, the programs should be adequate to ensure that all those "dids" and "did nots" are appropriate in light of whatever the prevailing standard is. This approach assumes, of course, that up-to-date, accurate, clearly communicated information about the standards is available to all facilities. Achieving this communication goal will be a significant challenge in many countries and it must precede the training and quality systems objectives if evaluations are to be meaningful.

FDA inspections

Before further exploring possibilities, the FDA inspection process will be briefly described to provide a common understanding of how USA inspections are currently managed.

Blood collection and component production facilities are required to register with the FDA. Every registered blood establishment is inspected annually by FDA district staff (investigators) trained both in inspection processes and requirements for blood establishments. In addition, facilities licensed to permit interstate shipment of blood products have a pre-licensure inspection in conjunction with the review and approval of their establishment and product licenses.

Both the pre-license and annual inspections determine if the firm is operating in accordance with cGMPs and other FDA requirements. Written documentation is an important part of demonstrating that FDA requirements are met and it is essential that comprehensive Standard Operating Procedures (SOPs) are consistently followed by all staff. Error and accident reports are specifically reviewed to ensure appropriate follow-up if there is an inadvertent release of products which fail to meet FDA requirements.

Checklists have been developed to identify major activities and key steps in blood bank operations [3]. Investigators use these checklists for a quick look at the operations and to report the general operations. The use of checklists helps ensure complete and consistent review of the wide range of manufacturing practices for the many different blood and blood component products processed in approximately 2400 blood facilities under FDA purview. Beyond the checklist questions, the FDA investigator determines what critical systems the blood bank uses to carry on its activities and selects some of the blood bank's system for coverage. For example, systems which include activities with an impact on HBsAg and HIV testing and related donor suitability decisions would usually be evaluated. The investigators review records, inquire about training and implementation, and make on-site observations to determine if the firm has adequate SOPs, competent personnel, and records to control its operations.

It is not generally practical for investigators to look at everything in a large blood bank. Thus, investigators may not review/assess all systems on any particular inspection, but overall, FDA inspections are very successful in identifying significant problems in blood establishments.

Quality Assurance guidelines

The recently published US Food and Drug Administration Draft Guideline for Quality Assurance in Blood Establishments (DGQABE, June 17, 1993) was developed through discussion at a public workshop which included participants from all sectors of the industry and several regulatory agencies [4, see Appendix I]. This document is intended to assist USA manufacturers in complying with cGMPs concerning all activities related to blood collection, processing, testing, storage and distribution. It is consistent with generally recognized principles of QA and it is meant to be used in conjunction with applicable Federal standards (regulations found in 21 DFR Parts 200, 211, 600-680 and 820) and FDA recommendations for blood establishments. This guidance (DGQABE) does not define specifically how standards are to be met, but rather identifies the need for comprehensive QA programs in every blood establishment, regardless of size. It defines the functions and responsibilities of the QA unit which will coordinate, facilitate and monitor all QA activities.

Each establishment in turn must develop its own specific SOPs to achieve the goals of: significantly decreasing errors; ensuring the credibility of test results; implementing effective manufacturing process and system controls; and, ensuring continued product safety and quality.

There is great flexibility which permits each facility to choose those approaches most suitable to its own circumstances, and the ways in which systems are designed to prevent, detect, investigate, assess and correct errors must be optimized for the specific situation. In future inspections of a facility which has established such QA systems, the most meaningful evaluation may be one which includes the assessment of the overall function of these systems rather than just the desired outcome, i.e., compliance with all applicable standards.

Blood establishments are expected to now have QA units which assure that well-written, accurate SOPs exist for every aspect of the operation; the SOPs must reflect validated processes and be implemented by personnel whose competency is appropriately documented by training, retraining and testing. All manufacturing should be conducted with properly qualified equipment in consistently controlled and monitored systems which are routinely audited. If systems meeting all of these criteria are in place for all of the key elements, one should find no deficiencies with respect to the requirements for blood establishments.

Future considerations for inspection models

If the type of inspection process changes, as with all new approaches to complex tasks, there will undoubtedly be an initial period where there is some decrease of efficiency because auditors will be reluctant to abandon tried and proven methods for the less familiar and superficially cumbersome "new" approach of looking at cross-cutting functions and control systems. Hypothetically, a novice could follow the detailed questions addressing all critical areas in checklists that currently form the backbone of most blood bank inspection programs. With the checklist in hand, one can ask the questions and record answers in the proper column even if one does not understand the concepts under review or their underlying principles. Perhaps one reason peer review evaluations have sometimes failed to detect serious problems is that less experienced inspectors may not adequately understand the interaction of complex systems involved in each situation. The more comprehensive systems approach ensures cGMPs will be met because the establishment has fulfilled their responsibility for proper system design as well as actively engaging the minds of workers in the ongoing tasks and multiple levels of decision-making in the complex milieu of 1990s blood establishments.

There is a huge potential for long-term gains in efficiency with a QA system review focus. Rather than looking at thousands of individual infectious disease marker test results, for example, and tracing many numbers of selected positive samples to demonstrate accuracy and proper follow-through in donor deferral lists, one might gain even more confidence that expectations for compliance with requirements are met if the facility can document: The effectiveness of those procedures and processes which are consistently used to achieve this goal, and; that training, competence evaluation and program oversight ensure that no deviations would have escaped notice in the facility's own internal audit program. As with all complex issues, there are many potential paths to the same endpoint, but it should be possible to define the expectations of standard-setting groups in ways that will yield to the challenge of developing better and faster ways to assess compliance.

One model might be constructed around a type of "self-audit" survey which is submitted in advance and includes off-site evaluation of detailed, written information concerning the control systems in place. This could be followed up with a much shorter on-site inspection to confirm truthfulness of the "self-audit" document and spot checking of each system's function, perhaps coupled with in-depth review of 1 or 2 key systems on a rotational basis.

From the standpoint of a regulatory agency's resource commitment to auditing, the 1992 average time spent for FDA inspection of a blood bank was approximately 30 hours per facility. The resource required to accomplish the approximate 2400 blood bank inspections was the equivalent of 78 full time staff positions for investigators and another 62 staff for administrative and technical support functions for the inspection program. If these values could be reduced by even 20 per cent without compromising the inspection effectiveness, the savings of resources (28 positions in the USA program) that could become available for higher priority concerns is obvious. The substitution of quality systems review for portions of the current inspection protocol presents a very important opportunity for resource reduction.

Not only might the on-site evaluation process become more cost effective, but it is generally recognized that quality systems planning and management are much more *durable* and effective measures that are less vulnerable to the individual human errors and accidents that cause even the "best" laboratories to occasionally suffer unexpected deficiencies. Without quality system planning and implementation, any record of past performance is only of historical value; with appropriate QA systems in place, however, one can predict that tomorrow's performance should continue at the established level or even improve.

The occasional discovery of misunderstood rules or system blind spots are potential hazards that can't be completely eliminated, and such problems may be more readily identified by an objective "outsider". Hence, most workers would agree that there are few substitutes for the kind of scrutiny a new observer brings to any review process. But, one can envision exchange "inspection" programs among similar size institutions supplementing the comprehensive quality system review process so effectively that the investigator may in the future detect system deficiencies only rarely because failures become rare. This potential elimination of lengthy inspections, and the resultant time-consuming documentation of deficiencies with pursuant enforcement action, could provide the opportunity for the regulatory authorities to focus on error-reduction research and to expand their role in training directed at good quality program design and implementation. Because some of the most significant errors occur rarely and randomly, it is not possible to do the needed error-reduction research in any one facility and coordinated national efforts are badly needed. Resources saved might also be devoted to improving the dissemination and understanding of information critical to compliance with both existing and new regulatory requirements.

By providing leadership in areas such as systems design and error reduction, the regulatory authorities may ultimately provide more benefit to the public health than spending the same amount of resources in repetitive inspections of existing systems that predictably fail because human error factors have not been reduced to the fullest extent possible.

In the USA we have taken the first step on the new pathway. The FDA has described the essential structure of QA programs in the recently released draft guideline and has provided lists of key elements related to each of several critical control points. This federal guidance is supplemented by the private sector's successful development of models for internal audit programs based on the same key areas. I would challenge each of you to contribute your ideas to the task which lies ahead in developing a new framework for external audit programs – one which will be derived from the new paradigms and which may be dramatically different. There is an essentially unlimited opportunity to explore ways to re-focus future attention of external audits to most effectively respond to the new levels of quality management that will exist in blood establishments. Let's save some of our creative energy for thinking about the external audit process in new ways and experimenting with approaches that have potential for increasing external audit effectiveness and efficiency.

Acknowledgement

The author gratefully acknowledges the valuable editorial assistance of Mr. Hector Zuazua and Mr. Jack Goodson, Division of Field Investigations, Office of Regulatory Affairs, FDA and Mr. P. Michael Dubinsky, Office of Compliance, Center of Biologics Evaluation and Research.

References

1. Title 21, Code of Federal Regulations, Parts 200, 211, 600-680, and 820. US Government Printing Office, Washington DC, 1993.
2. GMP for Blood Banks, Blood Transfusion Council of the Netherlands Red Cross. September 1992.
3. Form FDA 2609(5/91) Department of Health and Human Services (PHS), Food and Drug Administration Blood Bank Inspections Checklist and Report. Instruction Booklet for Blood Bank Inspection Checklist and Report.
4. Guideline for Quality Assurance in Blood Establishments. Rockville, MD. Food and Drug Administration, June 17, 1993. (Docket No. 91N-0450), Documents Management Branch (HFA-305), Food and Drug Administration, Rm. 1-23, 12420 Parklawn Dirve, Rockville, MD, 20857.

APPENDIX I

[DOCKET NO. 91N-0450]

DRAFT
Guideline for quality assurance in blood establishments
June 17, 1993

For further information about this document, contact:
Center for Biologics Evaluation and Research (HFM-635)
Food and Drug Administration
8800 Rockville Pike
Bethesda, MD 20892
301-295-9074

Submit written comments on this document to:
Dockets Management Branch (HFA-305)
Food and Drug Administration
Rm. 1-23
12420 Parklawn Dr.
Rockville, MD 20857

Submit requests for single copies of this document to:
Food and Drug Administration
1401 Rockville Pike
Rockville, MD 20852-1448
301-295-9000
Fax 301-295-8938

Comments and requests should be identified with the docket number found in brackets at the heading of this document.

Table of contents

Quality assurance in blood establishments

Purpose

The purpose of this guideline is to assist manufacturers of blood and blood components, including blood banks and plasmapheresis centers, in developing a Quality Assurance (QA) programme in their effort to be consistent with recognized principles of QA and current Good Manufacturing Practice (cGMP).

Scope

This guideline provides general information on procedures and practices and may be useful to blood establishments in developing and administering a QA programme. Because the Food and Drug Administration (FDA) is in the process of revising 21 CFR 10.90(b), this document is not being issued under the authority of 21 CFR 10.90(b), and the document, although called a guideline, does not bind the agency and does not create to confer any rights, privileges, or benefits for or on any person. Blood establishments may follow the guideline or may choose to use alternative procedures not provided in the guideline. If a blood establishment chooses to use alternative procedures, the establishment may wish to discuss the matter further with the agency to prevent expenditure of resource on activities that may be unacceptable to the FDA.

Blood and blood components applicable to the prevention, treatment, or cure of human diseases or injuries are biological products subject to regulation pursuant to Section 351 of the Public Health Service (PHS) Act [42 USC 262]. Similarly blood and blood components intended for use in the diagnosis, cure, mitigation, treatment, or prevention of diseases in humans are drugs and defined in Section 201(g) of the Federal Food, Drug, and Cosmetic (FD&C) Act [21 USC 321(g)]. Section 501(a)(2)(B) of the FD&C Act states, in part, that a drug shall be deemed to be adulterated if "the methods used in, or the facilities or controls used for, its manufacture, processing, packing, and holding do not conform to or are not operated or administered in conformity with cGMP to assure that such drug meets the requirements" of the FD&C Act. Because blood and blood components are drugs under the FD&C Act, the cGMP regulations in 21 CFR Parts 210 and 211 are applicable. In addition, FDA has issued cGMP regulations for blood and blood components in 21 CFR 606.

This guideline is intended to be used in conjunction with the applicable federal standards in 21 CFR Parts 600 through 680 and Parts 210 and 211. Section 210.2 provides that the regulations in Parts 210 through 226 and 600 through 680 are considered to supplement, not supersede, each other. Where it is impossible to comply with the applicable regulations in both Parts 210 through 226 and Parts 600 through 680, the regulations specifically applicable to the product shall apply and supersede the more general regulation. Some examples of 21 CFR Parts 210 and 211 and Parts 600 through 680 supplementing each other are set forth in Appendix A. This guideline may be amended periodically as needed.

Blood establishments should be aware that under the Clinical Laboratory Improvement Amendments of 1988 (CLIA), establishments performing laboratory testing, including blood banks and plasmapheresis centers, must also comply with applicable regulations in 42 CFR Part 493. These regulations, generally effective September 1, 1992, establish standards for laboratory personnel, quality control, proficiency testing, patient test management, and QA based on test complexity and patient risk factors.

Introduction

The United States has one of the safest blood supplies in the world. This is due in large part to the development and implementation of standards for donor suitability criteria and product quality. Since 1983, many significant developments have occurred including the implementation of new tests and donor suitability criteria. In addition, the FDA has intensified donor suitability criteria. In addition, the FDA has intensified its oversight of blood establishments and has documented the release of unsuitable blood and blood components in a number of situations due to deficiencies.

These findings may be related to several factors: The increase in the number of tests performed (increased testing increases the opportunity for errors and contributes to the complexity of the operation); the increasing use of complex advanced technology in testing procedures and equipment including computer systems; a shortage of appropriately trained health care and laboratory personnel; and the need for more sophisticated process and system control procedures in blood establishments, including procedures for training and supervising existing personnel.

In a memorandum dated April 6, 1988, FDA's Center for Biologics Evaluation and Research (CBER) requested that blood establishments review procedures and employee training programs to determine the adequacy of safeguards to prevent the release of unsuitable blood products. CBER issued a memorandum on March 20, 1991, notifying blood establishments of the increasing number of product recalls due to errors and accidents in manufacturing. CBER described examples of the types of errors and accidents that have resulted in the release of unsuitable products. In addition, CBER reminded establishments of the reporting requirement for errors and accidents and the need for follow-up investigation.

To ensure the continued safety of the nation's blood supply, it is essential that blood establishments implement effective control over manufacturing processes and systems. FDA believes that this can be accomplished by each blood establishment developing a well planned, written, and managed QA programme designed to recognize and prevent the cause of recurrent deficiencies in blood establishment performance. The goals of QA are to significantly decrease errors, ensure the credibility of test results, implement effective manufacturing process and system controls, and ensure continued product safety and quality. QA includes measures to prevent, detect, investigate, assess, and correct errors. The emphasis is on preventing errors rather than detecting them retrospectively.

Implementing a QA programme requires a commitment of time and resources. The design and scope of a QA programme depend on the size and complexity of manufacturing operations performed by the establishment. The potential public health consequences require that all establishments, regardless of size, invest in QA.

Quality control/Assurance programme

A QA programme is a system designed and implemented to ensure that manufacturing is consistently performed in such a way as to yield a product of consistent quality. QA is the sum of activities planned and performed to provide confidence that all systems and their elements that influence the quality of the product are functioning as expected and relied upon.

There are several dimensions to QA including quality control procedures and cGMP. Adequate quality control procedures are an element of conformity with cGMP and include the routine on-line or in-process monitoring of manufacturing procedures [See 21 CFR 211.22(a), 211.100(a)]. Other dimensions of QA relevant to the control of production include standards for personnel, facilities, procedures, equipment, testing and recordkeeping activities.

Quality assurance function

Title 21 of the CFR, Section 211.22(a) requires a quality control unit having the responsibility and authority to ensure product quality. In the pharmaceutical industry, the group performing this function often has been titled the Quality Control unit. With the evaluation of the concept of QA during the past 20 years, the group responsible for oversight of all activities relating to product quality (including quality control) often has been titled the Quality Assurance unit. Subsequently, in practice, the terms quality control often has been considered by many as limited to describing the component of a QA programme that includes the activities and controls used to determine the accuracy of the establishment's equipment and operations in manufacturing (i.e., on-line or in-process testing) and product release. Irrespective of the title of the person or persons performing QA duties, a quality assurance function should be established.

Although the term "quality assurance" is not used in 21 CFR Parts 210 and 211 and Parts 600 through 680, these regulations clearly require a programme of activities to control the manufacturing process to prevent the release of unsuitable products. For purposes of clarity, this document uses the term "quality assurance" to describe the actions, planned and performed, to provide confidence that all systems and elements that influence the quality of the product are working as expected. The person or group of persons who perform this function will be referred to as the QC/QA unit. The terms "quality control" and "quality assurance" will be defined as stated above and in the glossary.

The QC/QA unit should coordinate, monitor, and facilitate all QA activities. The QC/QA unit may include one or more individuals dedicated solely to QA functions or individuals who also perform other tasks in the establishment. In the latter situation, however, individuals should not have final oversight of their own work [See 21 CFR 606.100(c), 211.194]. In a small firm, it may be feasible for one individual to function as the QC/QA unit. That person has the responsibility for implementing controls and reviewing results of manufacturing to ensure that product quality standards are met.

Reporting responsibilities

A QC/QA unit should report to management or its designee. In licensed firms, this unit should report to the Responsible Head who is the individual designated in the establishment license application to represent the firm in its regulatory activities with FDA [See 21 CFR 600.10(a)] or his/her designee. In unlicensed firms, the QC/QA unit should report to a "designated qualified person" [See 21 CFR 606.20(a)] or his/her designee.

The Responsible Head or the designated qualified person is required to exercise control over the establishment in regard to all matters related to compliance with FDA requirements including the FD&C Act and the PHS Act, and should have the authority to implement corrective action when necessary. These individuals are responsible for ensuring corrective action has been taken. The Responsible Head or designated qualified person is also responsible for ensuring that personnel are appropriately assigned and trained to accomplish their duties [See 21 CFR 211.25, 600.10, 606.20].

The QC/QA unit reports independently from production to management. The QC/QA unit should ensure that production personnel follow cGMP. When necessary, the QC/QA unit should have the authority to stop production and/or release of product.

Quality control/Assurance unit responsibilities

The responsibilities of the QC/QA unit in blood establishments should include, but are not limited to, the following areas:

Standard Operating Procedures (SOPs) [See 21 CFR 211.100, 606.65(e), 606.100]

QA activities relevant to SOPs include:

(1) Determining that SOPs exist for all manufacturing procedures including, but not limited to, testing, and that SOPs accurately describe and define the procedure, including a statement of what the procedure is intended to accomplish. The actual content of the SOPs may be the responsibility of the production units [See 43 Federal Register (Fed.Reg.) 45014, 45032 Sept. 29, 1978].

(2) Reviewing and ensuring written approval of all SOPs prior to implementation and confirming that SOPs comply with all applicable statutory and regulatory requirements. Additionally, prior to the implementation of each SOP, the QC/QA unit ensures that the following items are written and in place:

(a) procedures to establish validation protocols to ensure that methods and processes accomplish their intended purpose;
(b) identification of personnel responsible for performing each procedure;
(c) procedures for training and certifying individuals identified in (b);
(d) responsibilities of supervisors for oversight of the performance of all procedures;
(e) methods for periodic proficiency testing;
(f) methods for periodic competency evaluation of the individuals performing each procedure;
(g) methods for evaluating the performance of each procedure during QA audits;
(h) designation of each procedure as a critical or non-critical control point (as defined in the glossary); and
(i) instructions for records maintenance consistent with requirements for record-keeping.

(3) Maintaining an index of all SOPs, a master copy, and an archive of obsolete SOPs.

(4) Ensuring that the SOP content is reviewed to assess impact on other systems and their functions.

(5) Ensuring that each employee is provided with, and has ongoing access to, the necessary SOPs to perform assigned duties.

(6) Ensuring that validation protocols are designed prospectively, performed and evaluated, and that written validation reports are prepared. Validation of a process already in use may be based upon accumulated production, testing and control data.

(7) Ensuring that modifications or changes in SOPs are appropriately documented including the rationale for the change. Ensuring that revised or new methods and processes are validated and do not create an adverse impact elsewhere in the system or operation. Changes in SOPs should be made in accordance with a written procedure and be formally approved before implementation.

(8) Ensuring that SOPs for all QC/QA unit activities exist and define the QC/QA unit's responsibility for performing SOP review, approval or authorization or, if appropriate, ensuring review, approval or authorization has been performed.

(9) Ensuring pertinent SOPs are promptly updated to reflect changes in manufacturer's directions for use and all SOPs are reviewed at least annually.

Training and education

The QC/QA unit should assist in developing, reviewing, and ensuring the approval of training and educational programmes for all personnel [See 21 CFR 211.25]. Training should include the following programmes:

New employee orientation;
cGMP training;
SOP training;
Technical training;

Supervisory training;
Managerial training;
QA training;
Computer training; and
Continuing education and training.

The QC/QA unit should be aware of factors that indicate a need for training or retraining. Information regarding the need for such training may be derived from management observations, proficiency test results, competency evaluations, technical changes, error/accident reports, complaints, QA audits, and problems discovered at critical control points identified in each system within the establishment's total operation. Thresholds for implementing retraining programmes should be established.

Competency evaluation

To ensure that all staff are trained and maintain their competency to perform all assigned tasks, the QC/QA unit should implement a formal regular competency evaluation programme. A competency evaluation programme should evaluate theoretical and practical knowledge of procedures including, but not limited to, the following:

(1) Direct observations of performance of routine and quality control procedures including, as applicable, donor suitability, sample handling, processing, testing, labelling, and instrument preventive maintenance;
(2) Monitoring the recording and reporting of test results by reviewing worksheets, quality control records, preventive maintenance records, and other records or computer entries;
(3) Written tests to assess problem solving skills, knowledge of SOPs, and theory; and
(4) Assessment of performance using internal blind specimens and external proficiency test specimens.

Minimum acceptable scores, performance, and remedial measures to correct inadequate performance on competency evaluations should be documented and retained in personnel records. Evaluation summaries provide useful information to correct individual or group performance problems.

Proficiency testing

Proficiency tests are commonly one part of the QA programme for testing laboratories. In addition to the facility's standard review of proficiency test results the QC/QA unit should also review, evaluate, and monitor the proficiency testing programme to ensure the adequate evaluation of test methods and equipment and competency of personnel performing testing.

Blood establishment proficiency testing procedures should ensure that proficiency samples are tested by all personnel normally performing routine testing, using routine test equipment, during routine test runs. Blood establishments should provide for proficiency testing of back-up or alternate test methods, e.g., manual procedures or "stat" tests. Procedures should ensure accurate, reliable, and prompt test results.

Supervisors, management, and the QC/QA unit should review and evaluate proficiency test results. Additionally, the QC/QA unit should analyze results for trends or patterns to identify specific problems. The QC/QA unit should also review, evaluate, and monitor the establishment's overall proficiency testing programme to ensure the adequacy of test methods and equipment, and competency of personnel performing testing. There should be a written plan for remedial action in the case of unsuccessful proficiency test performance.

Other quality control procedures may be useful in monitoring laboratory performance. These include statistical reviews of unknown and control sample results, comparisons of initial and repeat test values, and results of the same test performed by different methods or at different sites.

Validation

The FDA has provided general guidance in its *Guideline on General Principles of Process Validation* (May, 1987) which should be referenced to determine the validation principles applicable to an individual establishment's systems and processes. The QC/QA unit should ensure that adequate validation procedures have been performed. Complaints, errors, accidents, and problems at critical control points should be reviewed to determine the need for revalidation or revision of validation procedures.

Equipment

Equipment installation qualification is performed to establish "confidence that process equipment and ancillary systems are capable of consistently operating within established limits and tolerances" (*Guideline on General Principles of Process Validation*; May, 1987). The QC/QA unit should ensure that procedures are in place for equipment qualification, process validation, and revalidation after repairs to ensure the proper function of all equipment. Appropriate records of the results of validation testing should be reviewed and maintained.

There should be written procedures for equipment qualification, validation, maintenance, and monitoring. Additionally, there should be schedules for equipment monitoring, calibration, and maintenance sufficient to ensure that performance is according to specifications. Equipment monitoring procedures should include evaluation of consequences of malfunctioning or out-of-calibration equipment. Computer systems used in manufacturing are equipment subject to 21 CFR 211.68 and 606.60.

Error/Accident reports, complaints, and adverse reactions

The QA programme should provide assurance that procedures are in place and exactly followed for the review, evaluation, investigation, and correction of manufacturing errors and accidents. There should also be a system to ensure timely reporting to CBER of errors and accidents that may affect the safety, purity, or potency of blood products [See 21 CFR 600.14]. QA procedures should ensure that all complaints regarding product quality are investigated to determine whether the complaint is related to an error or accident in manufacturing. Investigative procedures should include provisions for review to determine whether the complaint represents an adverse reaction. Donor or recipient adverse reactions may be life-threatening, permanently disabling, or fatal. Procedures should be in place to ensure that donor and recipient adverse reactions are thoroughly investigated and completely documented. Facilities must be reported to CBER in accordance with 21 CFR 606.170(b). The QC/QA unit should ensure that product recalls and market withdrawals are handled according to established procedures and guidelines [See 21 CFR Part 7].

Procedures should be in place to ensure transfusion reactions are investigated. A programme should be in place to train patient care staff to recognize symptoms of adverse reactions so that appropriate intervention can be taken. Procedures should include review of manufacturing procedures when bacterial contamination of the product is suspected. Possible bacterial contamination should be reported to the blood collection facility.

An essential element of QA is feedback into the QA system of knowledge acquired through investigations of complaints, error/accident incidents, and adverse reactions. If there is no investigation of complaints, error/accidents, or adverse reactions, then factors contributing to the problems cannot be identified and corrected. Errors and accidents in manufacturing may be identified either by employees in the course of routine activities or by supervisors during record review. The QC/QA unit should assess all errors that occur during manufacturing, including those identified before products are released. The QC/QA unit should receive copies of error/accident reports and ensure appropriate follow-up actions have been taken. There should be procedures for initiating and completing all corrective actions. Corrective actions may include system redesign, retraining, and procedural changes.

Records management

The QC/QA unit should approve or ensure approval of all recordkeeping systems (manual and automated). Electronic or computerized recordkeeping systems should be properly validated [See 21 CFR 211.68]. QA procedures should be implemented to ensure that required records [See 21 CFR 606.160] are reviewed as necessary to ensure the accurate and complete history of all work performed. Portions of the review may be performed at appropriate periods during or after blood collecting, processing, compatibility testing, and storing [See 21 CFR 606.100(c)].

Lot release procedures

Each component (e.g., red blood cells, platelets, plasma, or cryoprecipitated AHF) prepared from a unit of whole blood represents one lot of product and bears a lot number, which is often the unit number assigned at the time of collection. QA procedures should be implemented to ensure that records are reviewed for accuracy , completeness, and compliance with established standards.

A second person should review each step in each process associated with every component prior to release [See 21 CFR 606.100(c), 211.194(a)(7)&(8)]. QA procedures should be in place to ensure that any lot discrepancies or failure of a lot or unit to meet its specifications are thoroughly investigated.

Labelling control procedures should be appropriate to the system and equipment. If automated labelling equipment retains information that could be erroneously printed during subsequent use, strict control procedures to prevent this should be implemented [See 21 CFR 211.125]. There should be written procedures designed and followed to ensure that correct labels, labelling, and packaging material are used for drug products [See 21 CFR 211.130].

Blood and blood components are labelled at various stages in the manufacturing process. At collection, products may be labelled as to the type of product the facility anticipates manufacturing. Products may be labelled as to blood group and expiration date at a later point in the manufacturing process. Products may be converted from one product type to another (e.g., fresh frozen plasma to recovered plasma, whole blood to red blood cells) and subsequently relabelled. Relabelling of blood products due to conversion to another product must undergo the same control procedures and have the same records maintained as the initial labelling operation.

At each stage in the manufacturing process where labelling occurs there should be process controls that ensure correct labels have been applied. Prior to release, the completely labelled product should be reviewed. Control procedures for final label review should include review of applicable production records and a record of verification by a second individual to ensure products have been properly labelled e.g., donor classification, blood group, expiration date, and product name. When proper control procedures for labelling are followed, labelling errors are minimized.

Quality assurance audits

A QA audit is one mechanism for evaluating the effectiveness of the total QA system. Comprehensive audits should be conducted periodically in accordance with written procedures [See 21 CFR 211.180(e)]. A comprehensive audit may consist of review of a statistically significant number of records. A focused audit may be necessary when quality problems have been identified, or to monitor, more effectively, a particularly critical area. However, isolated audits restricted to one area may not detect system-wide problems. The QC/QA unit's written procedures for a focused audit should be flexible enough to allow for additional audits without requiring changes in SOPs.

Audit procedures will vary in complexity depending on the size of the establishment and the specific processes under review. Individuals conducting audits should process sufficient knowledge, training, and experience to identify problems in the specific processes under review. The auditor or audit team should not be responsible for performing the procedures being audited. In situations in which an external audit programme is used, the QC/QA unit is responsible for assuring that the audit meets the needs of the establishment and is consistent with 211.180(e). There should be a written report documenting audit procedures and results. Procedures should include a plan for the Responsible Head or designated qualified person and other appropriate responsible officials to review and evaluate the results of the audit. The purpose of the review and evaluation is to ensure that responsible individuals are aware of problems, and corrective action is implemented. Audit reports should be retained consistent with product record retention requirements.

QA audits should be structured using a systems approach. Major systems of a blood manufacturing operation are identified in Tables 1-8, Appendix B. The systems which comprise blood establishment operations should include, at a minimum, the following:

Quality assurance;
Donor suitability;
Blood collection;
Component manufacturing;
Product testing;
Storage and distribution;
Lot release; and
Computer.

Each system may function independently or collectively with other systems. The critical control points in each system refer to areas that may affect the safety and quality of the product if key elements are not performed or functioning correctly. The key elements are individual steps in each critical control point. QA audits should evaluate critical control points and key elements in each system. Examples of critical control points and associated key elements are included in Tables 1-8, Appendix B. Each establishment should customize its audit for its own systems.

APPENDIX I.A

Examples of 21 CFR Parts 210 through 211 and Parts 600 through 680 supplementing each other

The cGMP regulations for drugs are crucial in ensuring the quality of blood and blood products and implementing these regulations is both feasible and practical. The cGMP regulations in 21 CFR 211 are general and suitable for all finished pharmaceuticals, and flexible to permit innovation. These regulations provide some flexibility to manufacturers to select the methods and processes most suitable for the products and operations of the individual firms. Notwithstanding such flexibility, manufacturers must, of course, create and implement procedures that are sufficient to accomplish all objectives of the cGMP regulations. In those few cases where precise procedures are set forth in the cGMP regulations, individuals believing that alternative mechanisms may also be acceptable are invited to request approval to use an alternative procedure pursuant to 21 CFR 640.120.

The term "lot" is defined for biological products in 21 CFR 600.3(x). This same term is also defined in 21 CFR 210.3(b)(10). The term "batch" is defined in 21 CFR 210.3(b)(2) as a specific quantity of a drug or other material that is intended to have uniform character and quality, within specified limits, and is produced according to a single manufacturing order during the same cycle of manufacture. For purposes of good manufacturing practice, a unit of whole blood or each of its components collected for transfusion or further manufacturing is both a lot and a batch. Testing for a single unit of blood may be performed as part of a run consisting of testing many other units of blood at the same time. In situations where testing (or other manufacturing) records include the results of more than one unit in a single record, signatures need only be written on the record as a whole rather that next to the results of each unit. The regulations in 21 CFR, Parts 210 through 226, and 600 through 680 are considered to supplement, not supersede, each other, unless the regulations explicitly provide otherwise. In the event that it is impossible to comply with all applicable regulations in both 21 CFR Parts 600 through 680 and Parts 200 through 211, the regulations specifically applicable to the drug in question shall supersede the more general regulations. The following charts provide examples of 21 CFR Part 211 and Parts 600 through 680 supplementing each other. The highlighted text in 21 CFR 211, cGMP for finished pharmaceutical, identifies additional standards of cGMP that are also applicable to blood and blood components.

Current Good Manufacturing Practice (cGMP) specific for blood and blood components	Current Good Manufacturing Practice (cGMP) for finished pharmaceutical (includes blood and blood components)
The biologic regulations describe requirements for record review, product quality control, laboratory controls, equipment controls, and SOPs for quality control, but do not explicitly refer to a QC/QA unit. The 211 cGMPs specify that a person or group of persons will be responsible for performing these functions [21 CFR 211.22]	211.22 (a) There shall be a quality control unit that shall have the responsibility and authority to approve or reject all components, drug product containers, closures, in-process material, packaging material, labelling, and drug products, and the authority to review production records to assure that no errors have occurred or, if errors have occurred, that they have been fully investigated. (c) The quality control unit shall have the responsibility for approving or rejecting all procedures or specifications impacting on the identity, strength, quality, and purity of the drug product. (d) The responsibilities and procedures applicable to the quality control unit shall be in writing; such written procedures shall be followed.
Comprehensive audit record review may consist of review of a sample of records that are representative of product production. A review of every complaint, recall and product failure must be performed.	211.180(e) Written records required by this part shall be maintained so that data therein can be used for evaluating, at least annually, the quality standards of each drug product to determine the need for changes in drug product specifications or manufacturing or control procedures. Written procedures shall be established and followed for such evaluations and shall include provisions for: (1) A review of every batch, whether approved or rejected, and, where applicable, records associated with the batch. (2) A review of complaints, recalls, returned or salvaged drug products, and investigations conducted under 211.192 for each drug product.

Current Good Manufacturing Practice (cGMP) specific for blood and blood components	**Current Good Manufacturing Practice (cGMP) for finished pharmaceutical (includes blood and blood components)**
606.100(b) Written standard operating procedures shall be maintained and shall include all steps to be followed in the collection, processing, compatibility testing, storage and distribution of blood and blood components for homologous transfusion, autologous transfusion and further manufacturing purposes. Such procedures shall be available to the personnel for use in the areas where the procedures are performed unless this is impractical.	211.100 (a) There shall be written procedures for production and process control designed to assure that the drug products have the identity, strength, quality, and purity they purport or are represented to possess. Such procedures shall include all requirements in this subpart. These written procedures, including any changes, shall be drafted, reviewed, and approved by the appropriate organizational units and reviewed and approved by the quality control unit. (b) Written production and process control procedures shall be followed in the execution of the various production and process control functions and shall be documented at the time of performance. Any deviation from the written procedure should be recorded and justified.
606.100(c) All records pertinent to the lot or unit maintained pursuant to these regulations (i.e., Parts 600 through 680) shall be rviewed before the release or distribution of a lot or unit of final product. The review or portions of the review may be performed at appropriate periods during or after blood collecting, processing, compatibility testing and storing. A thorough investigation, including the conclusions and follow-up, of any unexplained discrepancy or the failure of a lot or unit to meet any of its specifications shall be made and recorded.	211.192 All drug product production and control records, including those for packaging and labelling, shall be reviewed by the quality control unit to determine compliance with all established, approved written procedures before a batch is released or distributed. Any unexplained discrepancy ... or the failure of a batch or any of its components to meet any of its specifications shall be thoroughly investigated, whether or not the batch has already been distributed. The investigation shall extend to other batches of the same drug product and other drug products that may have been associated with the specific failure or discrepancy. A written record of the investigation shall be made and shall include the conclusions and follow-up.

Current Good Manufacturing Practice (cGMP) specific for blood and blood components	**Current Good Manufacturing Practice (cGMP) for finished pharmaceutical (includes blood and blood components)**
Record review specified in 211.192 may be performed by the QC/QA unit which is comprised of one or more individuals dedicated solely to QA functions or individuals who also perform other tasks in the establishment.	211.194(a) Laboratory records shall include complete data derived from all tests necessary to assure compliance with established specifications and standards including examinations and assays, as follows:
In the latter situation, however, individuals should not have final oversight of their own work. There should be SOPs describing product release procedures in emergency situations. Documentation of review of suitability of results included in in-process and laboratory testing records may consist of the signatures of the individual performing the procedure and the supervisor reviewing the records on the record as a whole rather than next to the results that pertain to the individual unit. Appropriate SOPs should be in place identifying individuals responsible for review and the criteria for review.	(7) The initials or signature of the person who performs each test and the date(s) the tests were performed. (8) The initials or signature of a second person showing that the original records have been reviewed for accuracy, completeness, and compliance with established standards.
	211.115 (a) Written procedures shall be established and followed prescribing a system for reprocessing batches that do not conform to standards or specifications and the steps to be taken to insure that the reprocessed batches will conform with all established standards, specifications, and characteristics. (b) Reprocessing shall not be performed without the review and approval of the quality control unit.

Current Good Manufacturing Practice (cGMP) specific for blood and blood components	Current Good Manufacturing Practice (cGMP) for finished pharmaceutical (includes blood and blood components)
606.20(b) The personnel responsible for the collection, processing, compatibility testing, storage or distribution of blood or blood components shall be adequate in number, educational background, training and experience, including professional training as necessary, or combination thereof, to assure competent performance of their assigned functions, and to ensure that the final product has the safety, purity, potency, identity and effectiveness it purports or is represented to possess. All personnel shall have capabilities commensurate with their assigned functions, a thorough understanding of the procedures or control operations they perform, the necessary training or experience, and adequate information concerning the application of pertinent functions of this part to their respective functions.	211.25(a) Each person engaged in the manufacture, processing, packing or holding shall have education, training, and experience, or any combination thereof, to enable that person to perform the assigned functions. Training shall be in the particular operations that the employee performs and in current good manufacturing practice (including the current good manufacturing regulations in this chapter and written procedures required by these regulations) as they relate to the employee's functions. Training in current good manufacturing practice shall be conducted by qualified individuals on a continuing basis and with sufficient frequency to assure that employees remain familiar with cGMP requirements applicable to them. (b) Each person responsible for supervising the manufacture, processing, packing, or holding of a drug product shall have the education, training, and experience or any combination thereof, to perform assigned functions in such a manner as to provide assurance that the drug product has the safety, identity, strength, quality and purity that it purports or is represented to possess. (c) There shall be an adequate number of qualified personnel to perform and supervise the manufacture, processing, packing or holding of each drug product.
606.20(c) Persons whose presence can adversely affect the safety and purity of the products shall be excluded from areas where the collection, processing, compatibility testing, storage or distribution of blood or blood components is conducted.	211.28 (a) Personnel engaged in the manufacture, processing, packing, or holding of a drug product shall wear clean clothing appropriate for the duties they perform. Protective apparel, such as head, face, and arm covering, shall be worn as necessary to protect drug products from contamination.

Current Good Manufacturing Practice (cGMP) specific for blood and blood components	**Current Good Manufacturing Practice (cGMP) for finished pharmaceutical (includes blood and blood components)**
In the Federal Register [40 FR 53534 Nov. 18, 1975], the Commissioner stated that the intent of this regulation is to also exclude from the processing area persons who may distract the attention of the personnel from the performance of their duties and persons who by their very presence in the processing area are capable of affecting the safety and purity of the product (e.g., persons moving from testing areas to the processing area without taking the necessary precautions.	(b) Personnel shall practice good sanitation and health habits. (c) Only personnel authorized by supervisory personnel shall enter those areas of the buildings and facilities designated as limited access. (d) Any person shown at any time (either by medical examination or supervisory observation) to have apparent illness or open lesions that may adversely affect the safety or quality of drug products shall be excluded from direct contact with components, drug products containers, closures, in-process materials, and drug products until the condition is corrected or determined by competent medical personnel not to jeopardize the safety or quality of drug products. All personnel shall be instructed to report to supervisory personnel any health conditions that may have an adverse effect on drug products.
The role of the responsible head in ensuring that personnel are appropriately trained and qualified for their duties is described in 606.10 and 606.20.	211.34 Consultants advising on the manufacture, processing, packing, or holding of drug products shall have sufficient education, training, and experience, or any combination thereof, to advise on the subject for which they are retained. Records shall be maintained stating the name, address, and qualifications of any consultants and the type of service they provide.
606.40(b) describes requirements for adequate ventilation. 211.46 describes ventiation control procedures in more detail.	211.46 (b) Equipment for adequate control over air pressure, micro-organisms, dust, humidity and temperature shall be provided when appropriate for the manufacture, processing, packing, or holding of a drug product.

Current Good Manufacturing Practice (cGMP) specific for blood and blood components	**Current Good Manufacturing Practice (cGMP) for finished pharmaceutical (includes blood and blood components)**
	(c) Air filtration systems, including prefilters and particulate matter air filters, shall be used when appropriate on air supplies to production areas. If air is recirculated to production areas, measures shall be taken to control recirculation of dust from production. In areas where air contamination occurs during production, there shall be adequate exhaust systems or other systems to control contaminants.
	211.48 (a) Potable water shall be supplied under continuous positive pressure in a plumbing system free of defects that could contribute contamination to any drug product ... (b) Drains shall be adequate size and, where connected directly to a sewer, shall provided with an air break or other mechanical device to prevent back-siphonage.
21 CFR 606.40(c) describes adequate, clean, and convenient handwashing facilities for personnel.	211.52 Adequate facilities shall be provided, including hot and cold water, soap or deter-gent, air dryers or single service towels, and clean toilet facilities easily accessible to working areas.
	211.68 (a) Automatic, mechanical, or electronic equipment or other types of equipment including computers, or related systems that will perform a function satisfactorily, may be used in the manufacture, processing, packing, and holding of a drug product. If such equipment is so used, it shall be calibrated, inspected, or checked according to a written programme designed to assure proper performance. Written records of those calibration checks and inspections shall be maintained. b) Appropriate controls shall be excercized over computer or related systems to assure that changes in matter production records or other records are instituted only

Current Good Manufacturing Practice (cGMP) specific for blood and blood components	**Current Good Manufacturing Practice (cGMP) for finished pharmaceutical (includes blood and blood components)**
	by authorized personnel. Input to and output from the computer or related system of formulas or other records or data shall be checked for accuracy. A backup file of data entered into the system shall be maintained except where certain data, such as calculations performed in connection with laboratory analysis, are eliminated by computerization or other automated processes. Hard copy or alternative systems, such as duplicates, tapes, microfilm designed to assure that backup data are exact and complete and that it is secure from alteration, inadvertent erasures, or loss shall be maintained.
606.40(d) Provide safe and sanitary disposal for the following: (1) Trash and items used during the collection, processing and compatibility testing of blood and blood products. (2) Blood and blood components not suitable for use or distribution.	211.56 (a) Any building used in the manufacture, processing, packing, or holding of a drug product shall be maintained in a clean and sanitary condition. Any such building shall be free of infestation by rodents, birds, insects and other vermin (other than laboratory animals). Trash and organic waste matter shall be held and disposed of in a timely and sanitary manner.
606.60 (a) Equipment use din the collection, processing, compatibility testing, storage and distribution of blood and blood components shall be maintained in a clean and orderly manner and located so as to facilitate cleaning and maintenance. The equipment shall be observed, standardized and calibrated on a regularly scheduled basis as prescribed in the SOP and shall perform in the manner for which it was designed so as to assure compliance with the official requirements prescribed in this chapter for blood and blood products.	211.67 (b) Written procedures shall be established and followed for cleaning and maintenance of equipment, including utensils, used in the manufacture, processing, packing, or holding of a drug product. These procedures shall include, but are not necessarily limited to the following: (1) Assignment of responsibility for cleaning and maintaining equipment; (2) Maintenance and cleaning schedules, including, where appropriate, sanitizing schedules; (3) A description in sufficient detail of the methods, equipment, and materials used in cleaning and maintenance operations, and the methods of disassembling equipment as necessary to assure proper cleaning and maintenance; ... (5) Protection of clean equipment from contamination prior to use; (6) Inspection of equipment for cleanliness immediately before use.

Current Good Manufacturing Practice (cGMP) specific for blood and blood components	**Current Good Manufacturing Practice (cGMP) for finished pharmaceutical (includes blood and blood components)**
	(c) Records shall be kept of maintenance, cleaning, sanitizing, and inspection as specified in 211.280 and 211.182.
606.100(b)(15) requires that SOPs include schedules and procedures for equipment maintenance and calibration. 606.100(b)(16) requires that written SOPs include labelling procedures and safeguards to avoid labelling mixups.	211.105 (b) Major equipment shall be identified by a distinctive identification number or code that shall be recorded in the batch production record to show specific equipment used in the manufacture of each batch of a drug product. In cases where only one particular type of equipment exists in a manufacturing facility, the name of the equipment may be used in lieu of a distinctive number or code.
606.120 (b) Labelling operation shall include the following controls: (1) Labels shall be held upon receipt, pending review and proofing against an approved final copy to ensure accuracy regarding identity, content, and conformity with the approved copy.	211.122 (a) There shall be written procedures describing in sufficient detail the receipt, identification, storage, handling, sampling, examination, and/or testing of labelling and packaging materials; such written procedures shall be followed. Labelling and packing materials shall be representatively sampled, and examined or tested upon receipt and before use in packing or labelling of a drug product. (b) Any labelling or packaging materials meeting appropriate written specifications may be approved and released for use. Any labelling or packaging that does not meet such specifications shall be rejected to prevent their use in operations for which they are unsuitable. (c) Records shall be maintained for each shipment received of each different labelling and packaging material indicating receipt, examination or testing and whether accepted or not ...

Current Good Manufacturing Practice (cGMP) specific for blood and blood components	**Current Good Manufacturing Practice (cGMP) for finished pharmaceutical (includes blood and blood components)**
606.100(b)(16) requires that written SOPs include labelling procedures and safeguards to avoid labelling mixups. 606.120 (b) The labelling operation shall include the following controls: (2) Each type of label representing different products shall be stored and maintained in a manner to prevent mixups, and stocks of obsolete labels shall be destroyed. (3) All necessary checks in labelling shall be utilized to prevent errors in translating test results. Label control procedures should be appropriate to control the specific labelling process or equipment. Procedures to reconcile labels should be performed if automated labelling equipment retains labelling information from previous runs that could be erroneously printed during the next use.	211.125 (a) Strict control shall be exercised over labelling issued for use in drug product labelling operations. (b) Labelling materials issued for a batch shall be carefully examined for identity conformity to the labelling specified in the master or batch production records. (c) Procedures shall be utilized to reconcile the quantities of labelling issued, used and returned, and shall require evaluation of discrepancies found between the quantity of drug product finished and the quantity of labelling issued when such discrepancies are outside narrow preset limits based on historical operation data. Such discrepancies shall be investigated in accordance with 211.192. (d) All excess labels bearing lot or control number shall be destroyed. (e) Returned labelling shall be maintained and stored in a manner to prevent mixups and provide proper identification. (f) Procedures shall be written describing in sufficient detail the control procedure employed for the issuance of labelling; such written procedure shall be followed.
Packaging is addressed in the 600 cGMPs in 606.65(a), pyrogen free container, 606.65(b), visual inspection, 606.100(b)(13), procedures to relate unit to donor, and 640.1(c), final container.	211.130 There shall be written procedures designed to assure that correct labels, labelling, packaging materials are used for drug products; such written procedures shall be followed. These procedures shall incorporate the following features:

Current Good Manufacturing Practice (cGMP) specific for blood and blood components	**Current Good Manufacturing Practice (cGMP) for finished pharmaceutical (includes blood and blood components)**
	(a) prevention of mixups and cross-contamination by physical or special separation for operations on other drug products. (b) Identification of the drug product with a lot or control number that permits determination of the history of the manufacture and control of the batch. (c) Examination of packaging and labelling materials for suitability and correctness before packaging operations, and documentation of such examination in the batch production record. (d) Inspection of the packaging and labelling facilities immediately before use to assure that all drug products have been removed from previous operations. Inspection shall also be made to assure that packaging and labelling materials not suitable for subsequent operations have been removed. Results of inspection shall be documented in the batch production records.
	211.134 (a) Packaged and labelled products shall be examine during operations to provide assurance that containers and packages in the lot have the correct label. (b) A representative sample of units shall be collected at the completion of finished operations and shall be visually examined for correct labelling. (c) Results of these examinations shall be recorded in the batch production or control record.

Current Good Manufacturing Practice (cGMP) specific for blood and blood components	**Current Good Manufacturing Practice (cGMP) for finished pharmaceutical (includes blood and blood components)**
606.40(a)(4) Quarantine storage of blood or blood components in designated location pending repetition of questionable serological results. 606.40(a)(6) Quarnatine storage, handling and disposition of products and reagents not suitable for use.	211.142 Written procedures describing warehousing of drug products shall be established and followed. They shall include: (a) Quarantine of drug products before release by the quality control unit. (b) Storage of drug products under appropriate conditions of temperature, humidity, light so that the identity, strength, quality, and purity of the drug products are affected.
Specifications and standards for blood, blood components, and products for further manufacture are outlined in the 600s. 606.140 Laboratory control procedures shall include: (a) The establishment of scientifically sound and appropriate specifications, standards and test procedures to assure that blood and blood components are safe, pure and potent and effective. (b) Adequate provisions for monitoring the reliability, accuracy, precision and performance of laboratory test procedures and instruments. (c) Adequate identification and handling of all test samples so that they relate to the specific unit of product being tested, or to its donor, or to the specific recipient, where applicable.	211.160 (a) The establishment of any specifications, standards, sampling plans, test procedures, or other laboratory control mechanisms required by this subpart, including any change in such specifications, standards, sampling plans, test procedures, or other laboratory control mechanisms, shall be drafted by the appropriate organizational unit and reviewed and approved by the quality control unit. The requirements in this subpart shall be followed and shall be documented at the time of performance. Any deviation from the written specifications, standards, sampling plans, test procedures, or other laboratory control mechanisms shall be recorded and justified. (b) Laboratory controls shall include the establishment of scientifically sound and appropriate specifications, standards, sampling plans, and test procedures designed to assure that components, drug product containers, closures, in-process materials, labelling, and drug products conform to appropriate standards of identity, strength, quality, and purity. Laboratory controls shall include: (1) Determination of conformance to appropriate written specifications for the acceptance of each lot within each shipment of components, drug product containers,

Current Good Manufacturing Practice (cGMP) specific for blood and blood components	**Current Good Manufacturing Practice (cGMP) for finished pharmaceutical (includes blood and blood components)**
606.60 (b) Equipment that shall be observed, standardized and calibrated with at least the following frequency, include but are not limited to: ...	closures, and labelling used in the manufacture, processing, packing, or holding of drug producs. The specifications shall include a description of the sampling and testing procedures used. Samples shall be representative and adequately identified. Such procedures shall also require appropriate retesting of any component, drug product container, or closure that is subject to deterioration ... (4) The calibration of instruments, apparatus, gauges, and recording devices at suitable intervals in accordance with an established written programme containing specific directions, schedules, limits for accuracy and precision, and provisions for remedial action in the event accuracy and/or precision limits are not met. Instruments, apparatus, gauges, and recording devices not meeting established specifications shall not be used.
Required and recommended viral marker testing, quality control testing, and other product testing combined with testing requirements outlined in an establishment's SOP are product specifications. Acceptance criteria are determined from product specifications.	211.165 (a) For each batch of drug product, there shall be appropriate laboratory determination of satisfactory conformance to final specifications for the drug product ... (d) Acceptance criteria for the sampling and testing conducted by the quality control unit shall be adequate to assure that batches of drug products meet each appropriate specification and appropriate statistical quality control criteria as a condition for their approval and release. The statistical quality control criteria shall include appropriate acceptance levels and/or appropriate rejection levels. (e) The accuracy, sensitivity, specificity, and reproducibility of test methods employed by the firm shall be established and documented ...

Current Good Manufacturing Practice (cGMP) specific for blood and blood components	**Current Good Manufacturing Practice (cGMP) for finished pharmaceutical (includes blood and blood components)**
	(f) Drug products failing to meet established standards or specifications and any other relevant quality control criteria shall be rejected. Reprocessing may be performed. Prior to acceptance and use, reprocessed material must meet appropriate standards, specifications, and any other relevant criteria.
606.120(a)(1) Labels shall be held upon receipt, pending review and proofing against an approved final copy, to ensure accuracy regarding identity, content, and conformity with the approved copy. 606.160(b)(2)(v) provides for maintaining records of labelling, including the initials of the person responsible.	211.184 (d) Documentation of the examination and review of labels and labelling for conformity with established specifications in accord with 211.122(c) and 211.130(c).
Master production and control records should include the signatures required in 211.186(a).	211.186 (a) To assure uniformity from batch to batch, master production and control records for each drug product, including each batch size thereof, shall be prepared, dated, and signed (full signature, handwritten) by one person and independently checked, dated, and signed by a second person. The preparation of master production and control records shall be described in a written procedure and such procedure shall be followed.
606.160(a),(b) describes recordkeeping requirements. Batch production records for blood and blood components need not be contained in a single record but should be easily traceable to document each significant step in manufacturing.	211.188 Batch production and control records shall be prepared for each batch of drug product produced and shall include complete information relating to the production and control of each batch. These records shall include:

Current Good Manufacturing Practice (cGMP) specific for blood and blood components	**Current Good Manufacturing Practice (cGMP) for finished pharmaceutical (includes blood and blood components)**
	(a) An accurate reproduction of the appropriate master record, checked for accuracy, dated and signed; (b) Documentation that each significant step in the manufacture, processing, packing, holding of the batch was accomplished, including:(1) Dates; (2) Identity of individial major equipment and lines used; (3) Specific identification of each batch of component or in-process material used; (4) Weights and measures of components used in the course of processing; (5) In-process and laboratory control results; (6) Inspection of the packaging and labelling area before and after use; (7) A statement of the actual yield and a statement of the theoretical yield at appropriate phase of processing; (8) Complete labelling control records, including specimens or copies of all labelling used; (9) Description of drug product containers and closures; (10) Any sampling performed; (11) Identification of the persons performing and directly supervising or checking of any significant step in the operation; (12) Any investigtion made according to 211.192; (13) Results of examinations made in accordance with 211.134.

APPENDIX I.B

Tables of systems

Table 1. System: Quality assurance.

Critical control point:	**QA unit established separately from production**
Key elements:	Objectives/policies Product specifications/validation Standard operating procedures Training in assigned duties/QA and cGMP for every employee Competency testing/proficiency testing cGMP/regulatory compliance Industry standards
Critical control point:	**Quality control**
Key elements:	Product testing Equipment testing Reagent testing
Critical control point:	**Audits**
Key elements:	System working separately and collectively Thresholds (limits) Alert levels/action levels Written audit reports Report evaluation/data analysis Feedback Corrective action/followup investigation
Critical control point:	**Complaints/defects/adverse reaction report evaluation**
Key elements:	Procedures include cause/effect evaluation Error and accident reports Laboratory error reports Donor callbacks User complaints Post transfusion disease ASAP evaluations Followup investigation/problem resolution
Critical control point:	**Information flow**
Key elements:	Regular review of manufacturer's instructions for use to identify changes and incorporate changes in SOPs Procdures to issue new/remove old SOPs Changes provided to actual users All shifts/backup personnel included FDA letters to those who need to know Managers receive accurate/timely information
Critical control point:	**Equipment maintenance/repair**
Key elements:	Validation/revalidation periodically or after repairs Preventative maintenance Routine/scheduled maintenance Maintenance records Qualification/validation after repair Repair records

Table 2. System: Donor suitability.

Critical control point:	**Donor recruitment**
Key elements:	Education
Critical control point:	**Donor registration**
Key elements:	Accurate information profided by the donor
	Accurate information entered in record files
	Certainty of identifiers/permanently effective
	Method to prevent known unsuitable donors from donating (example: Use of donor deferral registry at the time of registration)
	Record review
Critical control point:	**Donor screening**
Key elements:	Privacy
	Effective communication
	Consistent application of all health history and screening criteria
	Equipment/reagents
	Informed consent
	Quality control
	Record review
	AIDS education information/questions on high risk behaviour
	Donor medical history/donor medical examination
	Confidential unit exclusion (if performed)
Critical control point:	**Donor acceptance**
Key elements:	Acceptance criteria
	Documentation by authorized personnel/supervisory concurrence
Critical control point:	**Donor deferral registry (DDR)**
Key elements:	Accurate information/positive identification
	DDR availability at donation site
	Resolving discrepancies
	Changing information
	Adding/deleting information
	Identifying and resolving duplicate information
	Transferring information
	Record review
	Access to information
	Permanent vs. temporary conditions
	Data retrieval
Critical control point:	**Donor deferral**
Key elements:	Notification-donor/health authorities
	Additional testing
	Counselling
	Education
	Re-entry algorithm

Table 3. System: Blood collection.

Critical control point:	**Blood, component, source plasma collection**
Key elements:	Identification of donor, containers, pilot samples, components, records Verification that donor corresponds to container, pilot sample, components, records Arm preparation Equipment/supplies/IV solutions Collection set/container type Donor adverse reactions Overbleeding/underbleeding Product meeting specifications Automated collection Multiple component harvesting Volume of product retained/returned to donor Material defects Procedural errors Record review
Critical control point:	**Donor immunization programme**
Key elements:	Antigen safety, purity and potency Antigen selection and administration/schedules/doses Donor antibody production and evaluation Product specifications for labelled use/discard Disposition of low titer or other unsuitable product Donor medical record review Adverse reactions Product record review

Table 4. System: Component manufacturing.

Critical control point:	**Component preparation**
Key elements:	Acceptance criteria for source blood product (e.g. prolonged bleeds) Preparation time/temperature/equipment/weight or volume Assignment of expiration date Anticoagulant/additive solution/container Sterile connection device/pooling apparatus/other devices Record review Quality control (including sampling size) Disposition of all products Shipping, holding temperature Conditions of centrifugation Identification of personnel/equipment
Critical control point:	**Labelling manual**
Key elements:	Label acceptance review prior to use product specific expiration date assignment Verification of correct labelling Records of labelling operations

Critical control point:	**Labelling computerized**
Key elements:	Bar coding Label control, reconciliation On-line printing devices On demand/batch printing
Critical control point:	Quarantine
Key elements:	Location of product:untested, repeat test pending, biohazardous, not meeting specifications, unsuitable for transfusion, autologous, directed Processing record review/supervisory review Destruction or other disposition/records Equipment
Critical control point:	**Sterile connecting device**
Key elements:	Integrity of weld "Like tubing"

Table 5. System: Product testing.

Critical control point:	**Sample**
Key elements:	Identification/collection/labelling Integrity (dilution, contamination) Detection of missing samples/sample order Manufacturer's instructions/serum or plasma Storage time(s) and temperature(s) Records/sample acquisition Transportation conditions/transit time Retention of samples Disposal
Critical control point:	**Reagents**
Key elements:	Receipt records/transportation conditions Lot acceptance prior to testing/quarantine of untested materials Storage conditions and records Manufacturer's instructions for use Quality control testing/daily/acceptance of new stock Use of internal controls appropriate to assay/stability/reproducibility Records of errors or problems/reports to authorities
Critical control point:	**Equipment (including software, if appropriate)**
Key elements:	Intended use/design Interface compatibility (if appropriate) Qualification and calibration Maintenance and repair Training/introduction to new equipment Employee Validation Parallel testing Quality control Records Backup procedures Documentation of problems and reporting to FDA

Critical control point:	Laboratory testing
Key elements:	Sample identification/order/completeness Kit controls/data calculation/interpretation Reactive/positive test results/confirmatory testing Invalid tests/problems Repeat tests/test sequence Test interruption/start up/shut down/alternative methods Detection of missing test results Records Role of QA in release of test results Training/competency-based Proficiency testing

Table 6. System: Lot release.

Critical control point:	System: Lot release
Key elements:	Record review: All testing, required and recommended, was performed according to manufacturer's instructions and SOP and the results are acceptable for release Record review: All quality control was performed and results were within acceptable limits Record review: All manufacturing records verified and approved by designated, responsible personnel (supervisor) prior to the release of every component Record Review: Correct expiration date assigned Documentation of all review
Critical control point:	**Donor Suitability**
Key elements:	Record review Deferral registry

Table 7. System: Storage and distribution.

Critical control point:	Storage of products
Key elements:	Product location/place/order Products for further manufacturing Products quarantined (physical vs. computer) untested, repeat test pending, biohazardous, not meeting specifications, unsuitable for transfusion, autologous, directed Products availabe for distribution Products available for crossmatching Equipment Temperature Alarm system Record review
Critical control point:	**Distribution**
Key elements:	Record review Expiration date Visual inspection Packing/destination Validation of shipping containers Shipping temperature Records

Table 8. System: Computer

Critical control point:	**Documentation**
Key elements:	Hardware: Listing of components, installation date, serial numbers, maintenance records, electrical and environmental requirements, installation Software: Listing of programs, general program descriptions, program interaction, development, changes, archives, test plans, testing review and evaluation, and implementation date(s) Validation of components and systems Personnel/SOPs Training programs, outlines, and documentation
Critical control point:	**Testing the computer system**
Key elements:	Develop and maintain a test database/test scenarios (as appropriate) Develop and maintain test case protocols to cover normal, execeptional, boundary, stress, and invalid test cases Perform testing and document results Parallel testing Define and document evaluation of the test process Document modifications performed as a result of testing
Critical control point:	**Implementation**
Key elements:	Define and document implementation process Equipment interface Change control Approval process Procedures for backup and restore Procedures for data conversion(s) Procedures for downtime Software archives (as appropriate) Security/passwords
Critical control point:	**Maintenance**
Key elements:	Hardware Software for applications and operating systems Change control Approval process Archives Procedures for backup and restore Procedures for downtime Routine audits of data and systems

Also, please refer to the critical control points labelling-computerized, Table 4, Component manufacturing and equipment/software, Table 5, Product testing.

Glossary

Action Level: A limit determined by the QC/QA unit that indicates the need to immediately identify the source of an error and make the necessary corrections to avoid a compromise in product quality.

Alert Level: A limit determined by the QC/QA unit indicating that a potential problem needs to be identified and corrected but does not indicate that an affect on product quality has resulted.

Competency Evaluation: An internal process for assessing an individual's ability to perform all assigned tasks. A variety of performance appraisal methods may be used.

Computer Change Control: The process of identifying, evaluating, coordinating, implementing, documenting, and obtaining formal approval of changes in a computer system or database.

Critical Control Point: A function or an area in a manufacturing process or procedure that failure or loss of control may have an adverse affect on the quality of the finished product and may result in an unacceptable health risk.

Current Good Manufacturing Practice (cGMP): Methods used in, and the facilities or controls used for, the manufacture, processing, packing, or holding of a drug including, but not limited, to blood products to assure that such product meets the requirements of the FD&C Act as to satisfy and has the identity and strength, and meets the quality and purity characteristics, which it purports or is represented to possess. [FD&C Act, Sec.501(a)(2)(B)] cGMP ensures products are consistently manufactured and controlled by quality standards appropriate to their intended use. It encompasses both manufacturing and quality control procedures.

Key Element: An individual step in a critical control point of the manufacturing process.

Maintenance: Activities such as adjusting, cleaning, modifying, overhauling equipment to assure performance in accordance with requirements. Maintenance to a software system includes correcting software errors, adapting software to a new environment, or making enhancements to software.

Manufacture: Blood is produced by the body and requires further processing before it can be safely transfused. The term manufacture is defined, in part, in 600.3(u) as all steps in the propagation or manufacture and preparation of products. The biologics regulations prescribe requirements concerning all aspects of the manufacture of blood even before it is collected from the donor (e.g., donor suitability criteria). Manufacture is also used in the FD&C Act and the PHS Act in direct reference to blood and blood products [40 FR 53532, November 8, 1975].

Parallel Testing: Functional testing performed using two or more different systems simultaneously. This may include comparison of an established system to a new system. Parallel testing of a computer system(s) should include the use of actual data.

Production: The name given to personnel and/or operations involved in manufacturing.

Proficiency Testing: An evaluation of "the ability to perform laboratory procedures within acceptable limits of accuracy, through the analysis of unknown specimens distributed at periodic intervals by an external source" (Deboy and Jarboe, 1991).

Programme Description: A narrative that describes a computer programme's functions and interaction with other programmes.

Qualification: Establishing confidence that process equipment, reagents and ancillary systems are capable of consistently operating within established limits and tolerances. Process performance qualification is intended to establish confidence that the process is effective and reproducible.

Quality: Conformance of a product or process with pre-established specifications or standards.

Quality Assurance (QA): The actions, planned and performed, to provide confidence that all systems and elements that influence the quality of the product are working as expected individually and collectively.

Quality Assurance Audit: A documented independent inspection and review of a QA system, performed periodically according to written procedures to verify, by examination and evaluation of objective evidence, the degree of compliance with those elements of the QA programme under review.

Quality Assurance Programme: An organization's comprehensive system for manufacturing safe, effective, quality products according to regulatory standards. This programme includes preventing, detecting and correcting deficiencies that may compromise product quality.

Quality Control/Assurance QC/QA Unit: One or more individuals designated by, and reporting directly to, management with defined authority and responsibility to assure that all quality assurance policies are carried out in the organization.

Quality Control (QC): A component of a QA programme that includes the activities and controls used to determine the accuracy and reliability of the establishments' personnel, equipment, reagents and operations in the manufacturing of blood products including testing and product release.

Specification: Physical characteristics and composition, performance characteristics, parameters, requirements, standards, intended functions, behaviour or other characteristics of a product, system, or part of a system (as appropriate).

Test Cases: (as applied to computer systems)

Normal: valid data sets are used to produce normal outputs;

Exceptional: valid data which provide an unusual twist to force the programme to react to the unexpected;

Boundary: data which force the programme to evaluate conditions that are of borderline validity;

Stress: data which force the system to reach its maximum level of performance (during development and in the environment of the user);

Invalid: data that are not valid; test data should be designed to force a programme to prove that it can detect invalid input. Examples of invalid test cases may include an invalid donation date, e.g., 02/30/91; an invalid ABO group, e.g., "P"; a negative hemaglobin value; or no data entry.

Test Database: A database containing normal and abnormal values created by copying the production database and adding anomalous data. The test database is used to challenge a computer during validation and acceptance testing.

Thresholds: Guideline values which are needed in reviewing records to determine the adequacy of performance. These are the acceptable limits for quality to determine when intervention is necessary. Thresholds may be expressed as a number or percentage.

Validation: Establishing documented evidence which provides a high degree of assurance that a specific process will consistently produce a product meeting its predetermined specifications and quality attributes. A process is validated to evaluate the performance of a system with regard to its effectiveness based on intended use.

REFERENCES

Health and Human Services References

1. Title 21, Code of Federal Regulations, parts 210, 211, 600, 606, 610, 640, 660.
2. Center for Drugs and Biologics and Center for Devices and Radiological Health (CDRH), Guideline on General Principles of Process Validation (May, 1987).
3. FDA 91-4179: CDRH, Medical Device Good Manufacturing Practices Manual, 5th Edition (August, 1991).
4. FDA Compliance Program Guidance Manual, Blood and Blood Products, 7342.001 (1992), 7342.002 (1991).
5. FDA Compliance Policy Guide, FDA Access to Results of Quality Assurance Program Audits and Inspections, 7151.02, 1989.
6. FDA Memorandum: April 6, 1988, Control of Unsuitable Blood and Blood Components.
7. FDA Memorandum: March 20, 1991, Deficiencies Relating to the Manufacture of Blood and Blood Components.
8. Federal Register, Volume 43, No. 190, Friday September 29, 1978, Human and Veterinary Drugs, Current Good Manufacturing Practice in Manufacture, Processing, Packing or Holding, 45013-45087.
9. Federal Register, Volume 40, No 223, Tuesday, November 18, 1975, Human Blood and Blood Products, Collection, Storage and Processing, 53532-53544.
10. Federal Register, Volume 57, No. 40, Friday, February 28, 1992, Clinical laboratory Improvement Amendments of 1988; Final Rule, 7002-7288..

General References

Accreditation Manual for Hospitals, 1991, Joint Commission on Accreditation of Healthcare Organizations.

Bartlett R. Leadership for quality. ASM News 1991;57:15-21.

DeBoy J, Jarboe B. Government-mandated cytology proficiency testing: Practical, equitable and defensible standards. ORB 1993:152-61.

Juran J. Quality control handbook. McGraw-Hill, New York NY, 1994.

Kritchevsky S, Simmons B. Continuous quality improvement: Concepts and applications for physician care. JAMA 1991;266:1817-23.

Melum MM. Total quality management: Steps to success. Hospitals 1990;64(23):42,44.

Milakovich ME. Creating a total quality health care environment. Health Care Manage Rev 1991;16(2):9-20.

McLaughlin CP, Kaluzny AD. Total quality management in health: Making it work. Health Care Manage Rev 1990;15(3):7-14.

Olso A. Remmington's pharmaceutical sciences. Control 1980;16(82):1434-8.

Rosvoll R (ed). Accreditation requirements manual of the American Association of Blood Banks. American Association of Blood Banks, Arlington VA, 1990.

Walker R (ed). Technical manual. American Association of Blood Banks, Arlington VA, 1990.

BLOOD TRANSFUSION COMMITTEES AND OTHER APPROACHES TO IMPROVING CLINICAL TRANSFUSION PRACTICE

D.B.L. McClelland

In many countries, transfusion services now fall under the responsibility of national regulatory authorities concerned with the safety and efficacy of pharmaceutical products. As a result, many aspects of their work, especially those relating to the production of raw material plasma for fractionation, have been subject to regular inspection to ensure high standards of Quality Assurance (QA) and adherence to Good Manufacturing Practice (GMP). This regulation must be assumed to have made the products of the transfusion services both safer and better controlled in their adherence to nationally approved specifications such as the "Guidelines for blood transfusion services" in the United Kingdom [1].

While there is no doubt that substantial improvements will justifiably continue to be sought by national regulators, it is time to re-evaluate the gain to patient care likely to arise from this activity, and to examine other aspects of the transfusion process that so far have been subjected to little or no systematic or regulatory scrutiny. These include the prescribing of blood products, the whole clinical supply process (from blood bank to the patient's vein) and posttransfusion surveillance; possibly linked with studies on the influence of transfusion on short and longer term clinical outcomes.

Firstly, to turn to the prescribing of blood products, taking the example of red cells, we might usefully consider 3 problems.

1. There are existing clinical guidelines, deriving from consensus conferences and committees of wise men and women. However, it is unfortunately the case that the evidential basis for most guidelines is flimsy or absent. There are no randomized controlled clinical trials (RCCT) of red cell transfusion, although much animal work, and important clinical observations such as that on Jehovah's witnesses undergoing major surgery gives insights into critical thresholds for transfusion and a lot of recent work using non invasive monitoring methods is beginning to clarify the effects of hemodilution on the human myocardium.
2. Audit studies have repeatedly shown that guidelines are not adhered to (in fact many clinicians profess to be unaware of their existence or uninfluenced by them) [2].

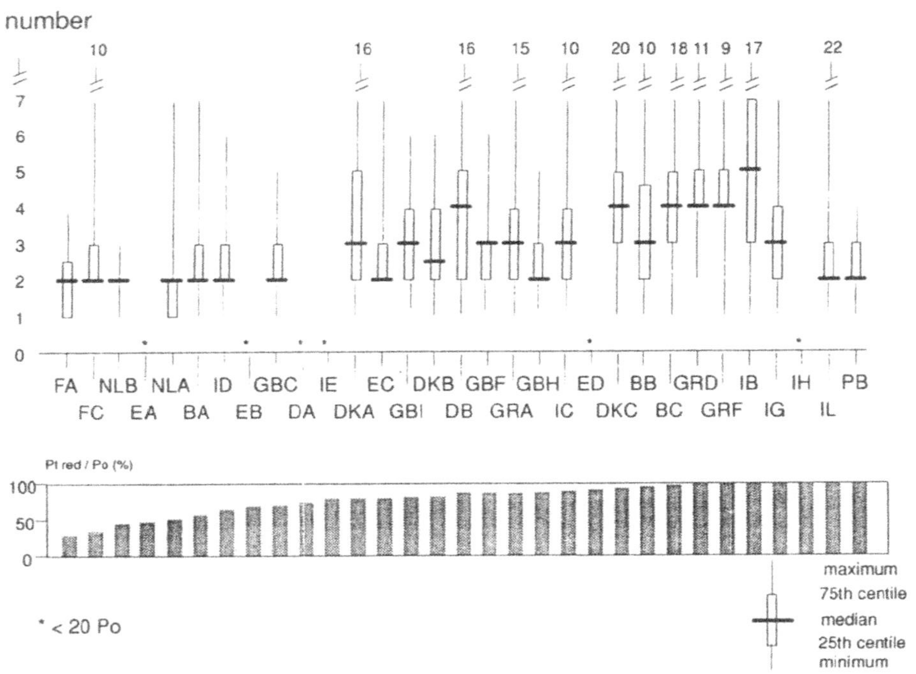

Figure 1. Variation in the use of red cells, albumin solutions and platelets in patients undergoing first time elective total hip replacement. Data from 28 European teaching hospitals. Pt/Po% = the percentage of all operated patients in each center receiving transfusion with each product. Data from SANGUIS Study [3].

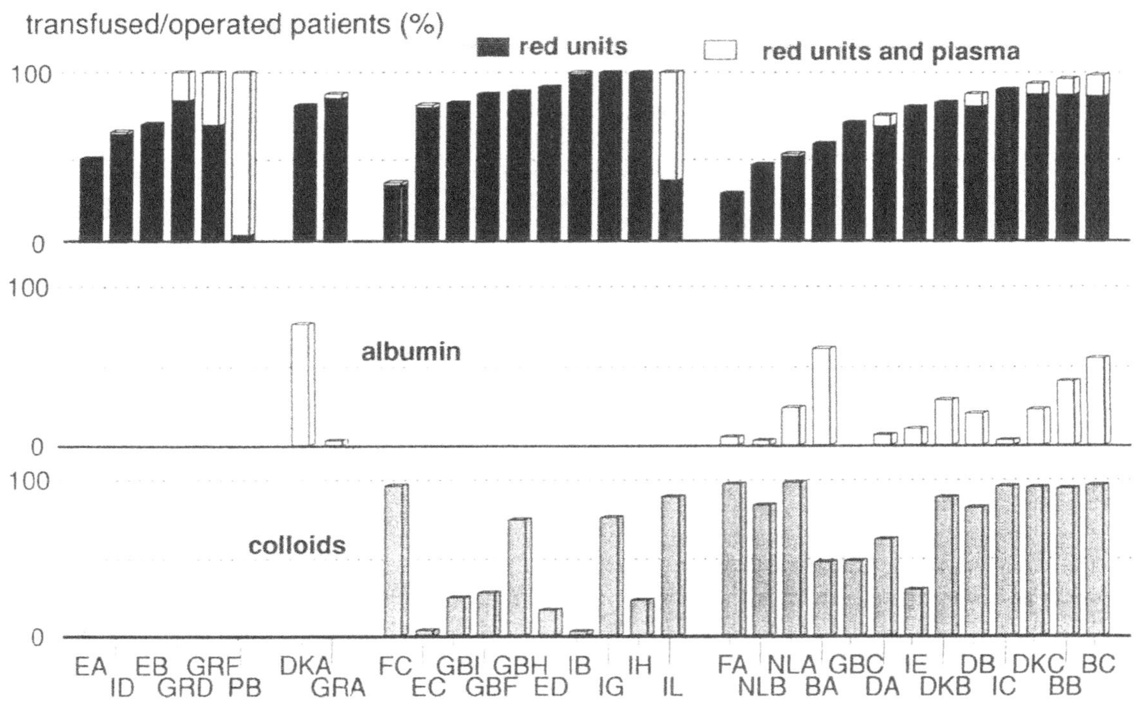

Figure 2. Variation in red cell use in patients undergoing first time elective total hip replacement. Data from 28 European teaching hospitals. Lower panel: the percentage of patients receiving any red cell transfusion. Upper panel: The number of red cell units received per patient transfused with any red cells. Data from the SANGUIS Study [3].

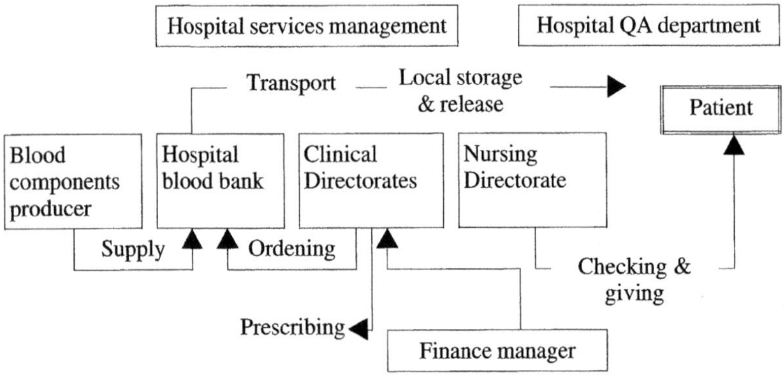

Figure 3 Who is responsible for managing the clinical transfusion process? Several different management structures are usually involved.

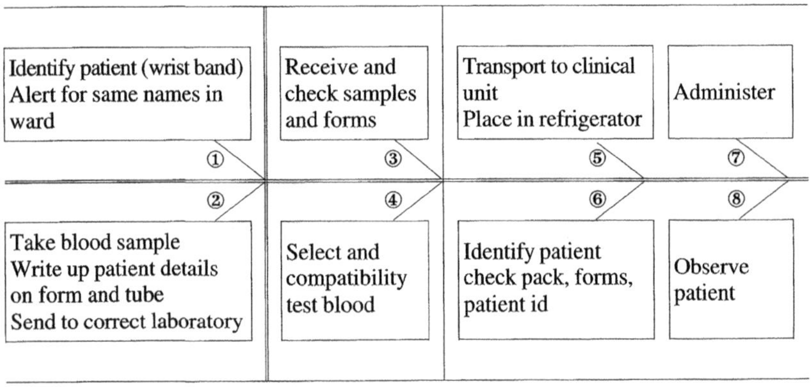

Figure 4. The clinical transfusion process is essentially linear (patient – blood bank – patient). A quality service will depend on a management system that takes responsibility for this process.

3. It is therefore perhaps not surprising that audit sutdies consistently reveal wide differences in red cell transfusion practice when well-standardized groups of patients are compared. Differences are marked in terms of the quantities of blood given and the post-operative hematocrit values that appear to be acceptable to different clinical teams. These are clearly illustrated in Figures 1 and 2 taken from the data of the SANGUIS study [3].

Clearly even in the absence of fully validated practice guidelines, these extremes cannot both represent optimal practice, and efforts to achieve more consistent adherence to what must currently be accepted as best practice must be a priority.

The second area of concern is what I wish to call the –clinical supply process". I have attempted to illustrate this simply in Figure 3 which illustrates the

Table 1. Evidence for weakness in the clinical sypply process.

- Ordering errors
- Sampling errors
- Prioritization failures
- Black holes in product life history
- Wrong blood incidents
- Near misses
- Poor recording

Table 2. Wrong blood given to patient: Minimum estimates.

- 1/29,000 RC units*
- Morbidity 1/275,00 0 units
- Mortality 1/550,000 unitts

111 identified in UK over 2 years

* UK 1992-3 McClelland & Phillips in press + Linden & Dressler 1992: 1/12,000.

organizational elements of the process leading from the withdrawal of a blood sample for matching, its transport and receipt by the blood bank, the testing, issue, transport and remote storage of the blood and its final administration to a patient (hopefully the one for whom it was intended).

A process diagram such as Figure 4 may illustrate more clearly the number of points at which things may go wrong, and evidence for such failures is provided by mishaps or uncertainties such as those summarized in Table 1.

If there is any doubt that all is not well, consider for example that in our own hospital over the past year, 5 per cent of all requests to the blood bank have a readily detectable error requiring corrective action, causing loss of integrity of the safety systems, and costing considerable personnel time not to say aggravation. More serious is the evidence for total system failures such as those described by Dr. Sazama in her chapter in this volume (pag. 35-43). Furthermore in a recent postal survey of all 400 blood banks in the UK, we obtained a 70 per cent response that enabled us to put minimum estimates on the frequency of these "wrong blood in patient" incidents [4]. Table 2 summarizes the findings and shows that our minimum estimate of 1/29,000 units going to the wrong patient is not dissimilar to the 1/12,000 figure estimated by Linden & Dressler on the basis of data from a mandatory error reporting system in New York [5]. A major contributor to these errors and a particularly sinister one for the blood banker, is the sample tube that is correctly labelled but contains the blood from the wrong patient. This is very difficult to ascertain. We made a minimum estimated of 1/6,000 samples but using double repeat blood grouping on separate samples from all patients, others have found a wrong blood in tube rate of 0.1 per cent.

The final symptom that I wish to mention of a poorly controlled process is the fact that despite our obsessive attention to maintaining the cold chain

Table 3. Management of improvement.

– Transfusion committees
– Hospital QA systems
– Nurse specialists
– Multi-disciplinary QI teams

Table 4. Composition of HTC.

– Clinicians from:
– anaesthesia
– intensive care
– surgery
– medicine
– pediatrics
– hematology
– oncology
– obstetrics
– Transfusion director and senior technical officer
– Nurse manager
– Junior doctor
– Medical records
– Hospital management
British Committee for Standardisation in Haematology, Transfusion Task Force.

throughout the blood components production process, most (perhaps all?) hospitals, are unable to provide strict documentation of the conditions in which blood units reside once they have been delivered to any remote refrigerator.

The potential for hazard due to storage of blood components in uncontrolled conditions must be high, when one compares this scenario with the rigorously controlled production processes. The problem belongs (whether they know it or not) to both clinical and non-clinical managers in the hospital and to individual clinicians carrying responsibility for the safe treatment of their patients. The challenge is to make things more secure – or in QA terms to bring the whole process under control. I suggest that the key features of a successful Quality Improvement (QI) program will include: awareness of the problem, audit to quantitate it, sound and *simple* procedures developed by or with the staff who actually do each part of the job, and continuing training for them. I doubt if strict regulation or enforcement approaches alone will achieve much. Fear makes the mistakes that occur go underground, disappear or pass unreported due to concern about retribution. Some of the approaches that may be effective are simply listed in Table 3.

First: The Hospital Transfusion Committee. A typical recommendation for the composition of an HTC is given in Table 4. The strengths of such a broad-based group are that it should have ample professional authority, and the wide range of QI activities that they may address are well documented in many publications on the role of the Hospital Transfusion Committee (HTC). However,

Table 5. Transfusion nurse specialist.

- Responsible to transfusion service
- Duty to ensure optimal transfusion care
- Works face to face with:
  - patients
  - clinical staff
  - blood bank
  - transport staff
- Establishes regular working relationships
- Conducts audit studies jointly planned by providers and user
- Training: informal and formal

Table 6. Transfusion nurse projects: Edinburgh 1993.

- Audit of patients' experiences of transfusion
- Analyse problems of patients dependent on red cell transfusion: implement individual care plans
- Home support of transfusion dependent patients
- Establish surgical bone harvesting: training of orthopedic teams, counselling of bone donors

I have reservations about the general practicability of this approach. Perhaps the greatest difficulty is assembling regular meetings of busy professionals for whom transfusion is not a prime interest but in reality represents a small element of the complex clinical interventions that they undertake daily. A wide survey of the participation in, and the proven achievements of HTC's would be of great interest but informal information suggests that many HTC's have problems in retaining active participation from key user clinicians.

A second real or potential problem is to define a clear and effective management process to "make it happen" when the HTC has decided on a course of action. Looking at Figure 3, it is, I suspect far from clear in many hospitals (certainly in the UK!), how one focuses the attention of the various management systems responsible for parts of the transfusion process to achieve an effective, coordinated process of decision and implementation.

My own prejudice is that we will only succeed in bringing this process under control if the transfusion service itself takes ownership of the problem and institutes effective action, of course consulting carefully with the relevant clinicians and managers. One way of moving in this direction is to appoint transfusion nurse specialists, based on the transfusion service but operating freely and with clinicians' support in clinical units. The main characteristics of this type of post are summarized in Table 5. Our experience has involved working with trained nurses experienced in a variety of clinical backgrounds (e.g. surgery, transplantation, community health), and usually appointed initially to undertake project work such as audit studies or development of tissue harvesting.

Table 6 illustrates some of the activities undertaken by these nurses in our region over the past two years. They have been instrumental not only in complet-

Table 7. Multi-disciplinary QI team method.

- Team analyses and maps the process
- Identifies 2 or 3 major weak points
- Devises action to improve
- Implements
- Monitors results against target
- Communicates findings
- Identifies further priorities

Table 8. Multi-disciplinary QI team: Edingburgh 1993.

- Customer survey showed ignorance of simple transfusion facts
- Action:
  - "Bloodfax" monthly information sheet
- Poor response times to emergency blood requests
- Action:
  - Retraining/education of laboratory team
  - Monitoring system installed
- Labels on packs hard to read in wards at night
- Action:
  - Change format, bigger clearer print
- No control on removal of blood from hospital refrigerator
- Action:
  - Pilot scheme with tamper-evident attachments
- Error rate 5% in submitted samples
- Action:
  - Set up error register. Use results in all teaching of medical students and house staff

ing specific audit projects but in establishing close contacts with patients and clinical staff and spontaneously becoming accepted as a natural source of informal training and problem-solving help in the clinical units. One of the most interesting projects has been a survey of patient's experiences of transfusion that has revealed how very poorly patients are informed about transfusion and how often their real concerns go unanswered during the episode of care [6].

An alternative, but complementary approach is to establish, ad hoc, a small multi-disciplinary QI team charged with improving a specific process. An example would be a team tasked with reducing errors or quality gaps in the hospital transfusion process: This could comprize a blood bank technologist, a clinical nurse, a junior doctor and the person responsible for blood deliveries. Their way of working need not be prescribed in detail but should include the steps shown in Table 7.

Examples of the activities undertaken by this type of informal group are given in Table 8. As with the nurses, this approach has "side benefits" beyond the specific remit, since the team is bound to come into contact and dialogue with clinical staff; this apparently simple step of improving contact between customer and provider can help to resolve many problems.

To guide and focus efforts on clinical quality improvement, a further useful approach is the user survey. A conventional questionnaire approach has proved highly informative in identifying areas of service in which clinicians perceived shortfalls that have been remedied only with significant change in attitudes and organization in our own service [7].

In conclusion

Quality improvement is fundamentally dependent on strong commitment from management – a top down element is vital. Management *must* support the QI team or the transfusion nurse with resources and lobbying skills when the necessary action has been identified. The patient focused transfusion nurse can be a highly effective trouble-shooter and trainer, does not threaten clinical staff and can work comfortably in a clinical setting as trainer, auditor and informal advisor. An effective and committed HTC will be a major asset in supporting and facilitating these approaches to quality improvement.

References

1. UKBTS/NIBSC Liaison Group. Guidelines for the blood transfusion service. 2nd edition. London: HMSO, 1993.
2. Salem-Schatz SR, Avorn J, Soumerai SB. Influence of clinical knowledge, organisational context, and practice style on transfusion decision making. Implications for practice change strategies. JAMA 1990;264:467-83.
3. SANGUIS Study Group. Use of blood products for elective surgery in 43 European hospitals. Full report to be published by EC May 1994.
4. McClelland DBL, Phillips P. Patients transfused with the wrong blood. A minimum of 111 incidents. Brit Med J 1994;308:1205-6.
5. Linden JV, Paul B, Dressler KP. A report of 104 transfusion errors in New York State. Transfusion 1992;32:601-6.
6. Giovanetti AM. Personal communication.
7. Gray S, Murphy W. A study of patients' percenptions and experience of blood transfusion. Scottish Med J 1994 (in press).
8. Pennington SJ, McClelland DBL, Murphy WG. Clinician's satisfaction with a hospital blood transfusion service: A marketing analysis of a monopoly supplier. Quality in Health Care; 1993;Vol II:239-42.

SCOTTISH NATIONAL BLOOD TRANSFUSION SERVICE

October 1993

BLOODFAX

**A monthly information sheet from Edinburgh and South-East Scotland Blood Transfusion Service.
Please circulate to your colleagues.**

Platelet Concentrates

Platelet concentrates are available in two forms. The first is prepared by centrifuging a unit of whole blood before it has been cooled for storage. The unit of platelets prepared in this way has a volume of about 50 mls and a platelet count of ≥55 x 10^9/l. A normal adult dose is 5 of these units and this would be expected to raise the platelet count by 30-40 x 10^9/l. The dose is scaled down for children - approximately 1 unit per 10 kg body weight. The second type of platelet concentrate is the apheresis unit. This is prepared by plateletpheresing a donor to give a unit which, in our region, has a volume of about 230 mls and a platelet content equivalent to 5 single units (ie a normal adult dose). In the South East Scotland Blood Transfusion Service most of our platelet concentrates are prepared from whole blood donations and the apheresis units are generally given to patients who have been shown to have poor responses to "standard" platelet concentrates or who are likely to need very frequent platelet transfusions.

Storage, Administration and Hazards of Platelet Concentrates

Platelets are stored at 22°C ("room temperature") for up to five days. They are stored on agitators as the platelets tend to stick together if they are not kept moving. Prior to issue the required number of units are generally pooled in one bag and as this is done by an "open" system the platelets must be given within six hours of pooling. The platelets should be given as soon as possible after reaching the ward and the transfusion should generally be completed within 30 minutes. If necessary they can be left at room temperature without agitation for a few hours but this should be avoided if possible. NEVER STORE PLATELETS IN THE REFRIGERATOR AS THIS WILL CAUSE FUNCTIONAL DAMAGE!

Apheresis units are prepared by a closed system and no pooling is needed - there is therefore no "six hour deadline" for this product. It has been shown that platelet concentrates maintain good function even if they have not been agitated for up to 24 hours. However, we do not recommend prolonged storage on the ward without agitation.

Give platelets through a standard blood transfusion set or platelet giving set with a 170 μm filter. Don't use a giving set which has already been used to give blood.

Platelet concentrates are not treated to destroy viruses and, because they are stored at room temperature bacteria can multiply. Although these risks are small this product should not be used unless clearly indicated. Remember that one adult dose will generally result in five donor exposures. Occasionally febrile or allergic reactions are seen. These are usually not severe but, when in doubt, STOP THE TRANSFUSION and consult the BTS Duty Doctor.

Some Indications for Platelet Transfusion

Bone marrow failure: After chemotherapy or radiotherapy, platelet transfusion may be necessary because of bleeding or to reduce the risk of bleeding in those with severe thrombocytopenia. There is still a great deal of debate about the appropriate threshold for the prophylactic use of platelets but a level of around 10 x 10^9/l has been suggested. Coagulation abnormalities, sepsis, invasive procedures, etc may increase the risk of bleeding and a higher threshold will be needed in these patients.

Platelet dysfunction: May be congenital or secondary to drugs (especially Aspirin, NSAIDs) uraemia or cardiopulmonary bypass surgery. Additional or alternative measures may be indicated in some of these patients (withdraw drug, raise Hb in uraemia, give DDAVP or cryoprecipitate). The bleeding tendency may be disproportionate to the platelet count.

Massive blood transfusion: Significant thrombocytopenia occurs after approximately 1.5 times the blood volume has been replaced but may occur sooner if the patient develops DIC (eg if shocked or severe tissue damage).

Prophylaxis for surgery: LPs, liver biopsy, laparotomy, etc requires a platelet count of >50 x 10^9/l. For critical sites such as brain and eyes a count of >100 x 10^9/l is indicated.

NEXT MONTH: How Do We Screen Our Donors?

COMMENTS/CRITICISMS TO: Dr Audrey Todd, Consultant, SEBTS, Tel: 031 229 2585 Ext 282

Figure 5.

DISCUSSION

T.F. Zuck and H.J.C. de Wit

T.F. Zuck (Cincinnati, OH, USA): Prof. Gormley, you talked earlier in your paper about inspection. Where does the inspection authority reside. The reason I ask this question is a rather important piece in terms of the legal relationship between the commission and the establishment.

L. Gormley (Groningen, NL): Current inspection is by the content authorities of the Member States at the moment. Most of the community legislation which demands inspection must be carried out in accordance with the principles of the subsidiaries by the competent national authorities.

H.J. Heiniger (Bern, CH): Mr. Hannema, as we all know there are certain Member States in the EC, which do presently not comply with the 89/381, especially not with the paragraph on voluntary, non-renumerated donors. How does the EC commission plan to enforce paragraph 3 and 4 of the 89/381.

H.I. Hannema (Amsterdam, NL): I think it is very difficult for the European Commission to do so. As I mentioned 35-50% of plasma is imported from paid donors. If the Commission tries to enforce it, those countries and they are mainly Spain, Italy, Portugal and Greece will be without their plasma products. So, in my view it will not be enforced.

K. Sazama (Sacramento, CA, USA): I would like to raise this question for all three persons: mr. Hannema, mrs. Hoppe and dr. McClelland. One concern that needs to be further discussed (and is often very troubling with regard to the regulatory environment in which we exist) is that there is frequently insufficient attention and/or resources devoted to training persons performing audits, particularly inspections. Mrs. Hoppe could you comment about how some of the savings that you projected might be devoted to looking serious at how best to train the regulatory persons charged with making determinations about compliance? Then, perhaps, mr. Hannema might comment about how training is accomplished in the European community and dr. McClelland in his hospital experiences.

P.A. Hoppe (Bethesda, VA, USA): Well I do not known that I have any solutions to offer. I think it is only logical that we have a quality assurance (QA) process for the way we do our regulatory business just as we expect blood banks to have a QA process. Certainly the training of personnel is a key item in any system. I do not have responsibility for training and it would be presumptuous for me to suggest how others are to go about it. I do think we can acknowledge that there is a responsibility to try to train staff as well as we can.

H.I. Hannema: I think that the management of human resources is very important. Mr. Bremer also said, that you have to have a people-oriented quality management. There are a few management tools to influence people and training is one of them. I think as we go on in time training and with other procedures to influence, human resources become more and more important.

D.B.L. McClelland (Edinburgh, UK): We have to put money into it. I would respond not just from the point of view of the hospital blood bank, but of the regional supplier center in the terms that we used earlier. We have not done very well until some two years ago. I think we are getting better. Our quality manager provides, as part of our operational plan, a continuing program of quality awareness for all staff. We have had, across the national service a program that is running slower than we would like, but it is running and sending key-staff to formal courses. The training of our top quality people in the regional centers has up to now been ad hoc two or three day courses on internal quality audit. It has become extremely evident to me and is now very much emphasized by this meeting, that we simply have to put a good deal more than a few days a year into training these key people. It includes center directors and managers in that over the next one or two years, to ensure that they really get top class training in GMP and/or inspection procedures. We have to invest in that. So, I think our position is we have a start, but I am realising increasingly that that start is quite inadequate. We have got to double or quadruple the time and cash input to that.

A. Heaton (San Francisco, CA, USA): I would like to make first of all the observation, that the quality assurance document mrs. Hoppe referred to is in many respects a very critical step forward, because it provides a guideline for those generating QA programs. Quality management is probably the single most critical program for a manager in blood center management at present.

I have a question for mr. Hannema: As one designs regulatory systems, it is very easy to design the outcome into the system. For example regulatory personnel are usually awarded and promoted for what they find. Consequently, when inspectors visit centers, if they do not find anything, then they are regarded as negligent. A good inspector always finds something wrong! That is hardly a dynamic that is desirable when a regulatory organization is created. In fact this has great potential to create conflict, because the investigator instead of being orientated towards helping the agency is rewarded only for finding something wrong or being critical of an organization. This is very much the case in the

United States where there are different sub-groups within the Food and Drug Administration (FDA). The Office of Regulatory Affairs which supervises inspections is separate from the Center for Biologics Evaluation and Research which sets the standards that the inspectors are supposed to use. Since the inspectors are not involved in setting the standards they make no attempt to help you since they are only there to find aberrations. So, my question to mr. Hannema is: If you have the freedom to design your system, what steps are you taking to try and build in into your regulatory inspection process a facilitatory aspect or an educational aspect to help people to design quality into their systems rather than to focus upon retrospective criticism of the failure to have sufficient quality.

H.I. Hannema: Well, you may be right for the United States, but I do not think if you are always right for the European community. A state civil servant does not always get rewarded for finding much. He can be promoted or whatever reward for not finding anything. I think he does not do his job well, if he does not give compliments. One of the human management tools is to make a compliment. If you do not find much tell them so. You will do much better and the blood bank will do much better, if you give them compliments. What you are actually raising as a question is: What will be the future of GMP, what will be the design of GMP ten years or twenty years from now. Well, that makes me philosophical. First, what we are doing now is the only thing we can do. We have a huge bureaucracy which is called GMP. We want to get rid of the bureaucracy, but how to do. I think the only way to do it is what mr. Bremer said: To get people oriented. I think in the United States the bureaucracy is even worse. The only way out is to get to human resources management, make compliments, get training. That is what I see will happen in the twenty years ahead.

A. Heaton: I would very much encourage you to use these workshop or consensus development meetings since they contribute toward QA rather than error management. It is an extremely useful process for helping an industry learn as it develops new approaches and allows the use of currently available experts to design quality into systems. Regulators can then use this information to improve on the systems as they conduct their inspections. One of our difficulties is that many of the investigators do not go through that process. They come from a totally different industry, the pharmaceutical industry. They then begin to apply rules that they have learned in a different industry, to the biologics industry. This can create great difficulties unless you design an educational process into your system.

D.B.L. McClelland: Don't you think that the ultimate test of performance of a regulatory system and its people should actually not be the finding of faults, but the quality of the whole operation. They should be like preventive medicine people. They should be paid for having really good healthy centers producing really good safe products.

P.A. Hoppe: I hope that the quality assurance document will help change the focus of inspections. I think if the operations improve in each center, the FDA is less likely to make long lists of the things that are wrong.

J.A. van der Does ('s-Gravenhage, NL): Dr. McClelland, unfortunatly I very much agree that it is very difficult to get transfusion committees in hospitals organized. In the Netherlands more than ten years ago we had a consensus development. There were about 500 doctors, all agreeing that it should be documented why you give a transfusion. We did a review in our area and none of the hospitals could provide data on why transfusions were given. You could get all the data about how transfusions were given, about what the hematocrits were, but there was no information on the doctor who decides what to give and why to give, documenting it and getting at the end the answer to the question "did you get what you wanted". So, the evaluation. You said, that a good hospital transfusion committee can sustain the nurse on the ward. What I think you are doing marvellously is getting around the doctors and I am starting to think that that is the only way to get in the hospital the right documentation: Not to try to educate the doctors, but to get around them.

D.B.L. McClelland: I am not sure what the question is, but I will respond to the comments. I have tried several times to get a transfusion committee together and I have never been able to get it to work. I think you are right, they do not work because people are too busy doing other things. That does make sense, because for us transfusion is a big thing, but for every clinician busy with patients the transfusion is just a small part of the total care process, that he and his team have to provide. All they want from transfusion is that they get the right blood in the right place at the right time. They want of course to establish a satisfactory platelet count the following morning or an adequate hematocrit and frankly as long as they get it, they are not going to waste time writing all that information down either. Neither of these things mean that they are bad doctors. It is just that they are busy doctors and certainly in the UK they are going to get busier and those problems are going to get worse. Secondly, I do not like the concept of getting round anybody in the clinical care team. I think that is a negative concept and I would not use it. I would put it another way. I think it is a matter of recognizing the jobs that are appropriate for certain people to do. If you have tried for five years having talked to 500 doctors and all of them saying that it is a good idea, and you go back and find that none of them have done what they agreed to, that is a very good experiment. To me it does not mean you have 500 bad doctors, it means that if that job has to be done it is just not going to be done by them, because it is forced down their priority list all the time by all of the other things they have to do. So, support them, do not go round them.

T.F. Zuck: In the United States there is a trend going on by the Joint Commission on Accreditation of Healthcare Organizations (JHO), in which they only recently are taking a very hard look at the operation of the transfusion service, which is now a requirement for the Joint Commission to accredit a hospital. I do not know whether this will effect physician's behaviour. It is very difficult to effect physician's behaviour. But if a hospital knows that it is going to lose its accreditation because it is deficient in this regard, I suspect that hospital management will have to take steps to assure that the charging is adequate, that the use of blood is appropriate. This is just emerging as an initial inspection and of interest by the Joint Commission.

C.Th. Smit Sibinga (Groningen, NL): To follow this up. I think what dr. Van der Does was saying is just a reflection of what happened over the past and is still ongoing. It happens in other countries as well. The point is that these 500 doctors who were in agreement with this consensus, went back to their place and did not find any support in their hospitals, no managerial support. That was basically the end of the story. Now we are in a different position. Mr. Hannema gave us a perspective of what is going to happen with respect to the hospitals in transfusion medicine. Secondly, we are in an economic recession period, in which the hospitals are forced to look more carefully at what they spend, which includes transfusion. We have seen in a number of our hospitals in the Northern region a mechanism in which suddenly one becomes more aware of the preciousness of transfusion and the need for evaluation. That is where the transfusion committees in our region now start to function differently to what they did in the past ten years. They were in place and functioning already ten years, but now something is happening. That is one comment.

I want to come back to the question of dr. Sazama. In the inspection and accreditation mechanism in the Netherlands, which was established in 1988, there is as a fundamental mechanism: An annual training for the inspectors, because we think that is a crucial point, not only in knowing precisely what to do and how to carry out an inspection, but also how to prevent conflict during an inspection.

A question to dr. Dumas. He spoke about the supplier and the manufacturer and quite rightly said the manufacturer should have some insight in what the supplier is actually doing in tracing back quality. But has he any thoughts about the reverse situation. Usually the supplier is supposed to receive back the finished products from the source material he is shipping over to the manufacturer. How about the supplier being involved in some kind of an audit of the manufacturer?

Y. Dumas (Maurepas, F): That is a very good question. That is not the situation today in the pharmaceutical industry, but I think that especially in Europe with the specific situation we have, this kind of relationship has to be largely developed. Today we are working with blood banks, who are providing plasma for fractionation, but also we manufacturers can be customers to them. So, I think it is a kind of relationship to be developed and in the future it must be an integral part of the overall QA system.

H.J.C. de Wit (Leeuwarden, NL): I was glad to hear that both mrs. Hoppe and mr. Hannema for the future are thinking of less bureaucratic systems then GMP tends to be now. We can see some differences in inspections of regulatory authorities between the United States and Europe. Could I ask them both how they see the near future, because what we hear about the United States is, that at this moment there is a lot of publicity around errors found in blood facilities, which gives a lot of concern even with donors about the safety of the blood supply. Small SOP deviations in a blood facility could lead to donors losing confidence and staying home, which might lead to a major quality problem.

P.A. Hoppe: I think that is a very good question, but one that is obviously difficult to comment on. The FDA enforcement strategy is one that comes from the highest levels of the FDA. The consideration of how much public information should be available is always a controversial question. The public usually wants to know, and they are not very able to balance their desire to know against the potential effect on the availability of blood or on other people's perception of the safety of blood. In some other areas such as nursing homes, the Health Care Finance Administration actually publishes a list showing who is good and bad. Again, you might question whether that is the right thing to do even when it is requested by the public. I think you are not likely to see any change in availability of information about problems in blood centers.

Y. Dumas: I would like to come back to a point that has been discussed. We feel that GMP is generating a big administrative workload. There are specific administrative people within fractionation centers, who do all the work that is required by the FDA or by the European Commission. We have to understand that it is an absolute necessity to take care of the process and for being able to react as quickly as possible to any deviation. But we should have a positive understanding that this is of help to us, to set up improvement step by step if we want to go to a better finished product at the end of the process. To achieve this we have to develop inside our structures positive thinking. This will require a lot of attention but it is achievable. I do not say this in the name of my company but in the name of people I am training at the university. We can achieve this very easily and we have to focus on people having a specific attention to communication in addition to having a good scientific background. Think positively and GMP will not be that much work to do.

D.B.L. McClelland: I would like to pick up the point that mr. De Wit has made. The ultimate quality issue for blood transfusion service is that it must demonstrate that a patient in its territory will never ever die of hemorrhage due to inadequate blood transfusion. There is no other primary quality requirement for a blood transfusion service but that. We have initiated a major debate about this in Edinburgh. If we do things or we fail to do things that affect the behaviour of the donors, such that they will discontinue to support the essential blood requirements, then all this talk about GMP is completely irrelevant, because we will fail our first and critical quality test.

A. Heaton: I think it is unfortunate, that this presentation has linked GMP with hospital transfusion committees, because in some respects they are at very different ends of the spectrum. The goal of GMP is to attempt to establish a product under standard specifications with minimum deviation and to generate a completely reproducible product in a documented fashion. That is what GMPs are attempting to achieve. With transfusion committees you are evaluating the performance of physicians who are trained to evaluate patients on the basis of the evidence they see in front of them, and to evaluate if they used their best judgement at the time of transfusion. While it may be appropriate to go back and make sure that clinicians did use their best medical judgement according to the latest facts, such review is very different to GMP. This review is QA and , whereas the former is good manufacturing practice. I believe that we should be careful to differentiate the two. We should never interfere with a clinician using his best clinical judgement, but of course, he should be subject to reasonable quality assurance review. At the manufacturing end, we should not be using good clinical judgement as we manufacture products, rather we should use manufacturing judgements and standards, so we produce the best products to the highest possible standards. There is a big difference between the two.

C.Th. Smit Sibinga: Dr. Heaton, that is exactly what the last session on Good Clinical Practice is going to inform us about!

III. Processing, Manufacturing and Quality Control Aspects

TEACHING AND TRAINING OF PERSONNEL: GOOD MANUFACTURING PRACTICES

T.A. Caglioti

Introduction

Good manufacturing practices require that each person involved in the manufacture of blood and blood components has the education, training, and experience to perform their assigned functions. One aspect of that training and education requires an adequate familiarity with the Good Manufacturing Practices (GMPs) that pertain to the assigned job duties. The blood banking industry is faced with not only the challenge of training to develop job-skill competencies, but also to satisfy the GMP performance demands. A comprehensive training strategy can not totally separate these two objectives, but instead should incorporate the relevant aspects of the GMP requirements into job-specific skill training.

The development of an effective GMP training program must utilize the established principles of instructional design used for any other area of training. The training process should be regarded as part of a dynamic *system* with components dedicated to the identification of operational requirements, design and validation of programs, trainer certification, outcome assessment and monitoring, and the establishment of feedback mechanisms allowing for program revisions and maintenance.

A summary of the steps involved in developing a GMP training program can be identified as follows:

1. Needs assessment.
2. Curriculum development.
3. Program development and validation.
4. Training implementation.
5. Assessing training efficacy.
6. Continuing GMP training.
7. Training documentation and administration.
8. Change control.

Though these steps are generic for any training activity, this article will focus upon their application towards the development of a training program that will satisfy the requirements of the GMPs

Needs assessment

The objective of needs assessment is to identify where training needs exist, and the knowledge, skills, and attitudes required to accomplish the work for which there is to be training [1]. This analysis starts at the organizational level, where the operational requirements are identified and then translated into the skill inventory necessary to satisfy these requirements. When developing a GMP training program, it is imperative that the organization has a clear understanding of all GMPs applicable to its operations.

The US Food and Drug Administration (FDA) has emphasized that the blood banking industry is subject to both the 200 and 600 series of the GMPs [2]. Contained in those requirements are also provisions for employee training. 21 CFR 211.25 *Current Good Manufacturing Practices for finished pharmaceuticals* (cGMPs), can be summarized as follows:

- Each person engaged in the manufacture of a drug product shall have the education, training, and experience to enable that person to perform the assigned functions.
- Training shall be in the particular operations that the employee performs *and in the current Good Manufacturing Practices (cGMPs) required by these regulations ... as they relate to the employees functions.*
- Training in cGMPs shall be conducted by qualified individuals on a continuing basis and with sufficient frequency to assure that employees remain familiar with the requirements applicable to them.

And from 21 CFR 606.20 *cGMP for blood and blood components:*

- The responsible head shall have the responsibility for assuring that employees are adequately trained in standard operating procedures and that they are aware of the application of the pertinent provisions of this chapter to their respective functions.

In a recent guideline "Quality assurance in blood establishments", FDA indicates that the Quality Assurance unit should also assist in the development, review, and approval of training programs for all personnel. These programs include the areas of GMPs, SOPs and technical training. From the regulatory perspective, the FDA expects industry to achieve GMP compliance through appropriate training in GMP awareness and in job skills.

Once the organization has clearly defined its operational requirements from a GMP perspective, the next step is to identify the skills requirement by the workforce to satisfy those requirements. This is done by performing a needs analysis, starting with an identification of the organization's current skill inventory. This skill-base is then compared to the skills identified when the operational requirements were defined. Usually, a "skill gap" becomes apparent, which is nothing more than the difference between skills *required* versus skills *existing*. One of the objectives of program development is to design training that will minimize or eliminate the skill gap.

The methods used in needs analysis include personal interviews, questionnaires, and performance observation. The analysis is usually conducted with the "top performers" for each job function and attempts to answer the questions of what skills are required for optimal performance of current and future task assignments. The needs analyst should then verify that the identified requirements support the objectives of the operational requirements identified at the corporate level.

Curriculum development

Once the training requirements are identified through the needs analysis, a training curriculum can be developed to satisfy those requirements. One trap that many firms fall into when structuring a GMP training program is the development of programs that simply reiterate the provisions of the regulations. This "page-turner" approach to GMP training usually serves only to further alienate this required topic from personnel.

Training in GMPs, as with most other training, requires some level of *awareness* training be given if personnel are ultimately expected to exhibit the new behaviour. GMP awareness training is designed to provide trainees with the history, scope, and *general* requirements of the regulations, so as to enable them to acquire the more specific application of GMPs to their job functions, received in subsequent training. Typical subjects for GMP awareness training may include the following:

- History and formation of the GMPs and regulating agency.
- Structure and authority of regulating agency.
- Application of GMPs to operations in your blood establishment.
- Structure of the regulations (21 CFR-GMPs, EC-GMPs, etc.).
- Inspection process and consequences of non-compliance.
- General requirements of the GMP elements: Record keeping, calibration, validation, Standard Operating Procedures (SOPs), etc. [4].
- Motivation/Incentive to individuals: Films, industry events, regulatory actions, etc.
- Periodic updates on new GMP requirements or operational vulnerabilities.

This awareness training should be provided to every employee of the blood center regardless of the extent of their direct involvement with manufacturing operations. The GMP provisions represent the minimum requirements for the manufacture of blood and blood components. It is not the FDA's intent to provide the specific details of *how* to comply with the regulations, but only to state *what* the requirements are. The GMP awareness training addressed this aspect of understanding the general requirements applicable to the organization. For example, almost all employees involved in the manufacture of a blood product will be documenting their performed tasks. Therefore, these employees need to be familiar with the GMP requirements for record keeping that describe how, when and where the FDA requires documentation to be accomplished. Once the general GMP concepts are established in the workforce, the next phase of training can move a step closer to the *execution* of the GMPs at the task level.

This next step of training will focus on *general* GMP requirements, but as they apply to discrete job functions. Personnel in the collection department may not need to familiar with 21 CFR 606.160 which states that "records be maintained for the visual inspection of whole blood and red blood cells during storage and immediately before distribution". This is a provision that is applicable to personnel in the storage and distribution operations and should be part of a GMP training program that addresses only those aspects of the GMPs that affect their assigned tasks.

In setting up the GMP training curriculum, this approach should be taken as a follow-up to the awareness training for each job function impacted by GMP requirements. To facilitate training, it may be possible to address multiple departments in a training session if the GMP requirements are common to all.

The final aspect of the training curriculum will focus on the incorporation of the GMP requirements into specific job-skill training. Using the above record keeping example, training for GMP compliance would be accomplished by providing the "how to" for the specific job task. In this case, documentation of visual inspection, trainees would be instructed on which form to complete, when, how, and what to do with the completed form. This further defines the general GMP requirement into required behaviours.

Since most job-skill training is derived from SOPs, this approach to GMP training can only be accomplished if SOPs are written to satisfy all necessary regulatory requirements. This is not to say that training in SOPs alone would be sufficient. At the very least, the skill training should be supplemented with the GMP awareness training and any other GMP training not addressed by the SOPs.

Program development

The development of GMP awareness training, both general and job-specific, involves an identification of the supplementary information that will instill a value and incentive for GMP compliance. Personnel working in regulated environments need to know *why* they have additional demands placed upon their performance. The reasons should go well beyond the traditional "because you *have* to ... it's the law". It's also helpful to provide a historical background of the regulation of the industry so that people can develop a frame of reference for the demands of these "external" requirements. Without a personal *value* for GMP compliance, a compliant operation will be very difficult to achieve. Hopefully, the value in blood establishment personnel will come from the realization that we need to assure the safety, purity, potency, and effectiveness of our products, and that each individual's job performance has the potential to affect those product attributes.

Performance-based training is focused on employee competency and specifies learning outcomes in operational behavioural terms. Specifying performance objectives involves the preparation of written statements that describe what the trainee is expected to do or demonstrate upon the conclusion of a training activity [5]. To establish these expected outcomes, one first needs to define the requirements of each job function down to the task level.

Task analysis details the skills required to produce a desired outcome. Each job function is usually made up of several tasks, each having a discernible output. The analysis is accomplished by conducting interviews with top performers, asking which skills are required to perform each task of their job. Task analysis can also be accomplished through written questionnaires or direct observation of job performance.

During the analysis process, it is important to maintain the focus on the GMP requirements affecting each task. It may be helpful if the interviewee prepares a list of all GMP provisions relevant to the tasks undergoing analysis, prior to the interview session. Such a list will help ensure that the GMP-associated behaviours will be integrated into the training program for each job function. The QA department should also be involved in the development process at this stage [3].

Program developers must verify, *during the development stage*, that all training programs are aligned with the operational objectives of the organization. The analyst needs to interpret all data in terms of what *needs* to be done, rather than perpetuate current performance with training that supports the required skills identified in the current task analysis alone. Changes in technology, equipment, regulatory requirements, customer demands, product attributes, or corporate quality pursuits, may all necessitate the acquisition of new skills in the workforce.

Once the needs and task analysis activities are completed, the developer should construct a content outline for the proposed training program and submit to appropriate department managers, subject matter experts, and QA for review. (The department managers may also wish to distribute the outline to representative staff members targeted for the training, for their review). This exercise represents the initial phase of program validation by allowing a technical review of the *program content*. There is no attempt to validate the efficacy of the program at this stage, instead the reviewers are asked to verify only if the training material is accurate. This is an opportunity for the developer to identify and correct major flaws in design of the program before implementation.

Training formats

In formatting GMP training programs, there are several training methodologies that may be considered for their suitability in achieving specific objectives. The following brief discussion includes some of the methodologies that have been used successfully in the quality engineering/GMP training program presented to blood establishments in the US [4].

– *Lecture*

The lecture format is the one most frequently abused in training programs – usually in its *overuse*. However, when used appropriately the lecture is valuable for the transfer of new concepts or technical knowledge. Appropriate lecturing allows for some group interaction at frequent intervals during the lecture. This can be in the form of questioning of participants, or periodically allowing the group to derive conclusions based upon the foregoing lecture. Prior to the start of any lecture, the participants should be encouraged to openly question or discuss the topics covered.

The lecture format is not appropriate when the training objective is the mastery of a skill, however, performance-based training offering hands-on practice is often *supplemented* by lecture.

– *Case studies*

The case study describes a problem situation to the trainees and then allows them to resolve the problem using the knowledge and skills presented in the training program. This methodology has been extremely effective when applied to GMP training. Case studies lend a sense of realism to the training and can stimulate genuine interest in the topics. Developers must construct the case studies to include several key learning points that they want the participants to derive from the case. During the actual implementation, the trainer must be careful not to disclose the learning points, but instead, to facilitate the group towards the resolution. Case studies can be written, video taped, or role played, with a list of key learning points provided to the trainer.

– *Workshops*

A workshop is just that: Participants will do some *work!* Workshops are the place for skill practice and mastery. The skill-acquisition objectives must be specified in advance so that the participants have an understanding of what they will be expected to *demonstrate* upon completion of the training.

In a GMP curriculum, there are definite skills that trainees will be required to exhibit in demonstrating that they can perform their job functions in a manner that satisfies the GMP requirements. These are the skills that were identified in the task analysis phase of the program development. Because skill-acquisition can be a time-consuming process, developers should limit the scope of each training module to a narrow, manageable set of skills.

– *Computer-based training (CBT)*

With increased computer assessibility and the development of simplified authoring software, computer-based training (CBT) is gaining in popularity. A recent survey of 2500 US corporations employing over 100 people showed that 58 per cent of them used CBT in their employee training [6].

CBT is excellent for transfer of theoretical and conceptual knowledge. With current graphics technology, rather than *lecture* someone on how blood products are irradiated, CBT can graphically display the theory, mechanics, and critical parameters of the irradiation process.

CBT does have a relatively high cost of program development, but that cost is diminishing as new software accelerates program development. In view of the development costs, CBT should be used for programs with a large enrolment and stable content. An appropriate application for CBT in GMP training would be in the development of a "Introduction to GMPs" program that could be used as part of the orientation for all new employees. For such an application, CBT is available 24 hours a day and can be run when any employee is ready for initial or refresher training.

– *On the job training*

On the job training (OJT) has earned questionable value as a training methodology because of its potential for lack of control and consistency in the content, quality, and delivery of training. This is an undeserved reputation attributable to poor program development and implementation, and not to any inherent aspect of OJT.

Like any other performance-based training, OJT must be structured with expected outcomes, course materials, and trainee evaluations, so as to minimize the potential for variability. OJT must take place in an environment that is supportive of learning, not in a "production line" atmosphere where efficiency is a primary concern. This hands-on training is a very effective method of providing supervised skill *practice*, and the trainee must not feel the pressure to perform perfectly from the onset.

Mentors involved in OJT will require adequate job function knowledge as well as training skills, allowing them to facilitate and evaluate the performance of the trainee. There is a need for continuous documentation of the trainee's progress in both the skill practice and any supplementary training. In situations where the process can not allow errors, e.g., an expensive product or component, adverse consequences of any error, etc., training must be performed on a simulated system that is as realistic as possible.

Implementation and validation of training

Once the training materials have been developed using appropriate formats, there should be an attempt to validate the training program, that is, *does the training program accomplish what it was designed to do?*

Validation of the program *content* was accomplished as described earlier at the end of the task analysis phase. As each training module is ready for implementation, there is a need to evaluate the impact of the training experience on employee performance. This can be done by first conducting a small group tryout on representative members of the target audience. A typical tryout group is 8-10 people of varied skill levels within the job area [1]. The training environment and presentation should be identical to routine training conditions. Upon completion of the tryout, the trainers should seek suggestions on how to improve the clarity, delivery, or effectiveness of the program. The program can then be revised if necessary.

The next phase of the program validation involves conducting the training under routine conditions, with the number of participants required by design. Once 50 or more people have completed the training, you can generate statistically significant data derived from post-training performance evaluations of the trainees. If the small group tryout was successful, there should not be a need for significant revisions to the program. If revision should be necessary, the validation process should be repeated starting with another tryout.

Assessing training efficacy

There are several tools that can be used in the short-term or immediate evaluation of GMP (or any other) training programs. A simple and direct measurement of knowledge transfer can be accomplished by administering a written knowledge-based test. If the identical evaluation is given before and after exposure to training, it can offer some evidence that the trainee has acquired new knowledge. These tests are appropriate for awareness training where there may be no demonstrable skills by which to evaluate performance.

When evaluating skill acquisition, the most direct method is that of performance observation. For job-skill training, trainees must demonstrate their skill mastery, including any GMP-associated behaviours addressed in the training program. The evaluators must be sure to assess the trainees *only* on their ability to execute the new skill correctly, not on their proficiency for the job requirements. Proficiency will develop with increased practice.

Another evaluative tool is to conduct interviews with the trainees after the training experience. Trainees are asked "What did you learn?" "Was it usable?" "... Valuable?", etc. If confidential responses are desired you can conduct the interviews using anonymous questionnaires. Trainees can then evaluate the total training experience: Content, usefulness, effectiveness, instructor capabilities, etc. Trainers and program developers should use the feedback to increase the quality and effectiveness of their programs.

The ultimate objective of training is to provide all personnel with the knowledge and skills required for the success of the organization. The short-term evaluations listed above do not provide adequate data for measuring the impact of a training program on the ongoing operations of the organization. For this information, performance evaluation needs to be done at a later period to assess if the training really has resulted in the desired performance of employees. In effect, this represents a long-term validation study of training efficacy.

The measurement tools are similar to those used in the immediate assessments. Interviews or questionnaires can be used with the trainees and with their managers. Managers should be questioned to see if there is a noticeable change in the performance of their staffs. To focus on GMP-related performance, data collected before and after training should be compared in areas capturing performance trends in GMP compliance (FDA inspection results), operational efficiencies, error/accident statistics, product failures, and the results of internal audits. If the results show that the training has not been as effective as anticipated, the evaluation should highlight the areas of the operation in need of additional training.

Continuing GMP training

The CFR requires that GMP training be conducted at a sufficient frequency to assure familiarity with the requirements applicable to one's job function [2]. Although the FDA can not specify what "sufficient frequency" means for all organizations, inspectors can evaluate if the current training schedule results in adequate familiarity with GMPs. This is accomplished during the inspection process through the observation of personnel practices, review of documentation, and the direct questioning of employees to assess their knowledge of GMPs.

Ongoing GMP training involves programs designed to reinforce or remediate personnel performance. Reinforcement training is a preventative measure against performance problems that involves planned and periodic reviews of the basic GMP concepts. These programs can be tailored to address job-specific GMP issues, as was done with the initial GMP training. This periodic training also offers the opportunity to instruct personnel on any minor changes to the requirements, or changes in the methods by which the requirements will be satisfied.

Remedial training is designed to correct unsatisfactory job performance. It requires identification of the cause for a specific non-compliance issue, and then attempts to eliminate the vulnerability through appropriate training. It is a common practice to "retrain employees in GMPs" after an operational deviation has occurred. In most cases the *reinforcement* aspect of additional GMP training is beneficial, but the real cause of the performance problem may lie outside the realm of GMPs.

The objective of continuous training is to maintain an awareness of GMPs in the workplace. This effort can be aided through the use of informal programs designed to keep GMPs "visible" in the organization. A GMP "newsletter" that depicts GMP related events from within the organization, industry, or related industries, can be an effective means of providing entertaining education to personnel. Posters, GMP contests, and the establishment of volunteer or rotational GMP audit teams can also be valuable.

Documentation of GMP training

Anyone working in a regulated industry is familiar with the unwritten edict concerning documentation: *If it isn't documented, it didn't happen.* This applies to all activities connected with training, from program development through implementation.

As stated earlier, all GMP training programs should be reviewed and approved by QA prior to implementation [3]. All details of the program should be included in an SOP that describes who gets trained, training frequency, qualification of instructors, how the training will be documented, etc. Full course descriptions should also be maintained for each training module that include a course content outline, module length, copies of any evaluations used, copies of all course materials, training methodologies used for delivery, and a history of any program revisions.

Documentation for any training session should include the course title or reference code that allows traceability back to the complete program documentation. Some form of attendance documentation should also be on file that includes the trainee name and signature, session date, start and finish times, and session instructor.

A data base can be developed that tracks all training for each employee and allows the generation of data sorted by various parameters. For instance, one could generate a list of all employees "certified" for a specific job function, or a list of all job functions for which any one employee has successfully completed the training. As discussed earlier, certification for any job function requires that the employee has also completed all required GMP training, including periodic refresher training. Such a data base can also serve to prompt required employee training through appropriate notification.

Change control

Once an organization has effective training systems in place, there needs to be a mechanism established to detect any changes that can impact the adequacy of those systems. The FDA has assigned a responsibility to the QA unit to "be aware of factors that indicate a need for training or retraining" [3]. Such indicators may include information derived from management observations, proficiency test results, competency evaluations, error reports, customer complaints, or internal audit findings. Many of these are operational indicators of an individual's performance degradation, but lend no clue as to the *reasons* for the performance change. These reasons may or may not indicate a training problem.

Performance problems in individuals that have been successfully trained and certified in job-skills should be evaluated from various perspectives. There may be a change in the individual's attitude and *willingness* to perform as required, most often resulting from personal problems unrelated to the immediate work activities. Changes in the employee benefit or compensation plan, increased workload, decrease or absence of personnel, or the introduction of new work requirements should all be considered during the evaluation.

The introduction of a new technology or a simple lack of skill practice due to infrequent task exposure are both causes for new or additional training activity. They also indicate a *system* problem in that people were being asked to perform functions for which they had inadequate or no training, and the situation was not being communicated to the individuals responsible for its remediation. Additionally, all personnel should be trained to report when their skill level is inadequate for an assigned task, without fear of punitive actions resulting from their self-reporting [5].

Summary

Increased testing, regulatory requirements, customer demands, and the introduction of new technologies will continue to place additional demands on the training programs of the blood banking and related healthcare industries. The FDA and accrediting agencies will remain steadfast in the requirement that each employee have the education and training necessary to accomplish their assigned functions.

It is important that top management demonstrate a real commitment to training and convey it as an activity critical for the success of the business. This is especially true for GMP training, where it can be easily indicated that the only reason the company provides the training is because it's an FDA or Health Authority requirement. If the employees receive that message there will be no personal value instilled for good manufacturing practices, and the organization will be vulnerable to compliance problems.

A comprehensive GMP training program should consist of both general awareness and performance-based job-skill training. Effective training will allow personnel to make appropriate, quality-based decisions when facing new and different scenarios during the execution of their assigned tasks.

References

1. Mayo GD, DuBois PH. The complete book of training: Theories, principles, and techniques. University Associates, Inc., San Diego, CA, 1987.
2. Code of Federal Regulations, Title 21 – Food and Drugs. Part 211, Current Good Manufacutring Practices for Finished Pharmaceuticals: 211.25.
3. Food and Drug Administration, Center for Biologics Evaluation and Research. Draft Guideline for Quality Assurance in Blood Establishments. June 17, 1993.
4. Ortho Diagnostic Systems Inc., Council of Community Blood Centers. Quality Engineering/GMP – Train the Trainer Program. 2nd ed. 1993.
5. Levchuk JW. Training for GMPs. J Parent Sc Tech 1991;45:270-5.
6. Training (ed). 1993 Industry Report. October 1993;30:29-34.

GOOD MANUFACTURING PRACTICE IN TRANSFUSION MEDICINE: JOB DESCRIPTIONS AND STANDARD OPERATING PROCEDURES

B.T. Teague

Like many of my colleagues, I concur our profession has dramatically changed. While some of this change has produced some beneficial results, I am somewhat concerned that the majority of the change has not increased the safety of the blood transfusion and has placed the cost of providing the service out of control.

To illustrate this point, we will take a brief look at The Blood Center in Houston, Texas, which represents a large regional blood center in the United States. The Center began operations in January of 1975 with a staff of 63 professionals, collected 46,000 units of whole blood, had an annual budget of USD 1.1 million, provided services to patients in about 80 hospitals in a 15,000 square mile area, and the service fee on a unit of red blood cells was USD 35. Because of substantial increases in several areas (patient needs, increased testing, inordinate bureaucracy, etc.) we have had to grow rapidly. Today, our staff numbers over 430, we collect about 185,000 whole blood units, plus over 20,000 apheresis procedures, our budget now exceeds USD 32 million, we serve over 130 health care facilities, and patients in these facilities will use about 500,000 units of blood and blood components. The service fee on a unit of red blood cells is now USD 70.

Our greatest challenge has not been keeping up with the medical and technical aspects of this growth, but rather the administration and management aspects. Additionally, the general public and the governmental agencies seem much more interested in the administrative and management aspects than the medical/technical ones.

We will take a look at some of the components of job descriptions, Standard Operating Procedures (SOPs), the Quality Control (QC)/Quality Assurance (QA) program, and how the current Good Manufacturing Practices (cGMP) are integrated into each.

Additionally, and probably equally important, we will take a look at how an organization can effectively provide leadership to implement these changes and discuss the difference between leadership and management.

In the United States, the Food and Drug Administration (FDA) has the responsibility for oversight of blood establishments, including the regulation, inspection and enforcement areas. These regulations are outlined in a "Code of

Federal Regulations" (CFR). As has been indicated by previous speakers, the primary resources for blood banks are 21 CFR 200 through 299 [1], 21 CFR 600 through 799 [2], and 42 CFR 493.

21 CFR 211.22(a) [1:82] requires that a QC unit has the responsibility and authority to insure product quality. Although the term "quality assurance" is not used in 21 CFR 210 and 211 and 600 through 680, these regulations clearly require "a program of activities to control the manufacturing process to prevent the release of unsuitable products" [3]. The QC/QA unit should coordinate, monitor and facilitate all QA activities. For example, at our blood center, the "Quality Assurance/Compliance Officer" heads our QC/QA unit and reports to the Chief Executive Officer as responsible head. This reporting responsibility is critical! The unit must report independently from production to management and should insure that production personnel follow the cGMP.

The position description should include the authority to stop production and/or release a product and oversight of SOPs. Additionally, the QC/QA unit should assist in developing, reviewing and insuring the approval of training and educational programs for all personnel (21 CFR 211.25) [1:82]. Training should include the following programs:

- New employee orientation.
- cGMP training.
- SOP training.
- Technical training.
- Supervisory training.
- Managerial training.
- QA training.
- Computer training; and
- Continuing education training.

The position description should also include the responsibility to be aware of factors that indicate a need for training or retraining. This information can be obtained from management observations, proficiency test results, competency evaluations, technical changes, error/accident reports, complaints, QA audits, and problems discovered at critical control points. The position description should also include thresholds for implementing retraining programs and competency evaluation, if so indicated.

SOPs (21 CFR 211.100 [1:88], 606.65 [2:30] and 606.100 [2:30] should include QA activities relevant to each SOP. For example, SOPs should exist for all manufacturing procedures including, but not limited to, testing, and accurately describe and define the procedure, including a statement of what the procedure is intended to accomplish. The actual content of the SOP may be the responsibility of the production units. Additionally, the SOP should include responsibility for reviewing and insuring written approval of all SOPs prior to implementation and confirming that SOPs comply with all applicable statutory and regulatory requirements. Also, prior to the implementation of each SOP, the QC/QA unit insures the following items are written and in place:

1. Procedures to establish validation protocol to insure that methods and processes accomplish their intended purpose.
2. Identification of personnel responsible for performing each procedure.
3. Procedures for training and certifying individuals identified in item 2 above.
4. Responsibilities of supervisors for oversight of the performance of all procedures.
5. Methods for periodic proficiency testing.
6. Methods for periodic competency evaluation of the individuals performing each procedure.
7. Methods for evaluating the performance of each procedure during QA audits.
8. The designation of each procedure as a critical or non-critical control point.
9. Instructions for records maintenance consistent with requirements for record keeping.

The QC/QA unit should ensure that the following processes are completed following implementation:

1. An index of all SOPs, a master copy and an archive of obsolete SOPs should be maintained.
2. The SOP content should be reviewed to assess impact on other systems and their functions.
3. Each employee should be provided with, and have ongoing access to, the necessary SOPs to perform assigned duties.
4. Ensure validation protocol are designed prospectively, performed and evaluated, and that written validation reports are prepared. Validation of a process already in use may be based upon accumulated production, testing and control data.
5. Modifications or changes in SOPs are appropriately documented including the rationale for the change. Ensure that revised or new methods and processes are validated and do not create an adverse impact elsewhere in the system or operation. Changes in SOPs should be made in accordance with written procedure and be formally approved before implementation.
6. Ensure that SOPs for all QC/QA unit activities exist and define the QC/QA unit's responsibility for performing SOP review, approval or authorization or, if appropriate ensure review, approval or authorization has been performed.
7. Ensure pertinent SOPs are promptly updated to reflect changes in manufacturer's directions for use and all SOPs are reviewed at least annually.

Each person engaged in the manufacture, processing, packing or holding shall have education, training and experience, or any combination thereof, to enable that person to perform the assigned functions. Training shall be in the particular operations that the employee performs and in cGMP (including cGMP regulations and written procedures required) as they relate to the employee' functions.

Training in cGMP shall be conducted by qualified individuals on a continuing basis and with sufficient frequency to assure that employees remain familiar with cGMP requirements applicable to them.

Each person responsible for superfixing the manufacture, processing, packing or holding of a drug product shall have the education, training and experience, or any combination thereof, to perform assigned functions in such a manner as to provide assurance that the drug product has the safety, identity, strength, quality and purity that it purports or is represented to possess.

There shall be an adequate number of qualified personnel to perform and supervise the manufacture, processing, packing or holding of each drug product.

It is important to understand the bias in all this "good manufacturing practice" dialogue. First, it is important to continue to believe the provision of blood and blood components constitutes a service and not a product. One simply cannot believe you can take something as precious as human blood and label it a product which would give it the same status as an air conditioner, automobile or a tank.

These comments should not be misinterpreted. Although there is total support for the provision of blood and blood components in the safest manner reasonably possible, there are, however, concerns that the continued reference to blood banking as a pharmaceutical industry and to blood as a product will denigrate the service and reflect very poorly on the donor public who so generously and unselfishly gives blood.

Having said that, the reality in our profession is that it has changed. Those of us who have recognized the change and accommodated it will continue to provide services. Those who, for whatever reason, do not change will find another profession or vocation, because they will not survive.

Now that we know what is needed in the change, how will you and your organization get the needed changes implemented? Take an informal survey in your own organization and ask this question, "How will we get from where we are to fully implementing needed changes in our organization?" The guess is that you will get several responses, including references to leadership, management, spend some money, and many more. The two most commonly heard references are "leadership and management". It has also been my experience that most people use these two words interchangeably and feel they both mean pretty much the same thing. The fact is they are not only not the same, but are substantially different.

What we call management is largely the product of the last 100 years and a response to one of the most significant developments of the 20th century: The emergence of large numbers of complex organizations. Modern management was invested, in a sense, to help the new railroads, steelmills, and automobile manufacturers achieve what legendary entrepreneurs created them for. Without such management, these complex enterprises tended to become chaotic in ways that threatened their existence. Good management brought a degree of order and consistency to key dimensions like the quality and profitability of products.

In the past century, literally thousands of managers, consultants and management educators have developed and refined the processes which make up the core of modern management. These processes, summarized briefly, involve the following:

1. Planning and budgetting: Setting targets or goals for the future, typically for the next month or year; establishing detailed steps for achieving those targets, steps that might include timetables and guidelines; and then allocating resources to accomplish those plans.
2. Organizing and staffing: Establishing an organizational structure and set of jobs for accomplishing plan requirements, staff and jobs with qualified individuals, communicating the plan to those people, delegating responsibility for carrying out the plan, and establishing systems to monitor implementation.
3. Controlling and problem solving: Monitoring results versus plan in some detail, both formally and informally, by means of reports, meetings, etc.; identifying deviations, which are usually called "problems", and then planning and organizing to solve the problems.

These processes produce a degree of consistency and order. Unfortunately, they can produce order on dimensions as meaningless as the size of the typeface on an executive memoranda. But, that was never the intent of the pioneers who invented modern management! *They created management to help keep a complex organization on time and on budget.* That has been and still is its primary function.

Leadership is very different. It does not produce consistency and order, as the work itself implies, it produces movement. Throughout the ages, individuals who have been seen as leaders have created change, sometimes for the better and sometimes not. They have done so in a variety of ways, though their actions often seem to boil down to establishing where a group of people should go, getting them lined up in that direction and committed to movement, and then energizing them to overcome the inevitable obstacles they will overcome along the way.

What constitutes good leadership has been a subject of debate of centuries. In general, we usually label leadership "good" or "effective" when it moves people to a place in which they and those who depend upon them are genuinely better off, and when it does so without trampling on the rights of others. The function implicit in this belief is instructive or adaptive change.

Leadership within a complex organization achieves this function through these subprocesses which can briefly be described as follows:

1. Establishing direction: Developing a vision of the future, often the distant future, along with strategies for producing the changes needed to achieve that vision.
2. Aligning people: Communicating direction to those whose cooperation may be needed so as to create coalitions that understand the vision and that are committed to its achievement.
3. Motivating and inspiring: Keeping people moving in the right direction despite major political, bureaucratic and resource barriers to change by appealing to the very basic, but often untapped, human needs, values and emotions.

Management and leadership, so defined, are clearly in some ways similar. They both involve deciding what needs to be done, creating networks of people and relationships that can accomplish an agenda, and then trying to insure that those people actually get the job done.

They are both, in this sense, complete action systems; neither is simply one aspect of the other. People who think of management as being the only implementation part of leadership ignore the fact that leadership has its own implementation process – aligning people to new directions and then inspiring them to make it happen. Similarly, people who think of leadership as the only part of the implementation aspect of management ignore the direction-setting aspect of leadership.

Leadership by itself never keeps an operation on time and on budget year after year. Management by itself never creates significant useful change. They are both needed if organizations are to fulfil their missions. In John Kotter's *A force for change: How leadership differs from management* [4], he strongly suggests that most firms today have insufficient leadership and are "over-managed" and "under-led" [4:10]. As we look at the cGMP and all that it entails, we would be wise to listen to Kotter very carefully.

Clearly, leadership and management will be sorely needed. It is leadership that will produce change. That is its primary function. In cases of effective leadership, the direction of that change will be carefully selected in an activity that is at the core of what leadership is all about. To understand that activity, it is absolutely essential to recognize what it is not. Setting direction is never the same as planning or long-term planning, although people regularly confuse the two. Planning is a management process, fundamentally deductive in nature, and primarily designed to help produce orderly results, not change. This is quite different from the direction-setting aspect of leadership and is directly applicable to the implementation of cGMP.

Good planning is incredibly important in organizations today. Our profession is complicated because of the number of people involved and the interdependence of activities that, without good planning, commitments to patients, donors and staff will go unmet, with all the inherent problems that tend to follow. Without good planning, organizations have a tendency to lurch from one crisis to the next, exhausting people, resources and funds in the process. If we are to implement cGMP successfully, we must want to be the best at what we do. This notion of wanting to be the best is a far more important theme in successful efforts than most people realize. It is always connected to a sensible strategy or set of strategies, but again and again, it is there. One of the challenges we have in transfusion medicine is that the best may not be good enough when the public and/or governmental agencies expect zero defects and/or pure safety when such is not possible.

In summary, the safety of the blood supply continues to be a primary concern for all of us in transfusion medicine. The development and implementation of standards for donor suitability criteria and product quality have substantially improved this safety. To insure the continued safety of the blood supply, it is essential that effective control over manufacturing processes and systems be implemented. The FDA believes this can be accomplished by each blood establishment developing a well-planned, written and managed QA program designed to recognize and prevent the causes of recurrent deficiencies in blood establishment performance.

The goals of the QA program are to significantly reduce errors, insure the credibility of test results, implement effective manufacturing processes and systems controls, and ensure continued product safety and quality. These efforts should include measures to prevent, detect, investigate, assess and correct errors, with the emphasis on preventing errors rather than detecting them retrospectively.

Implementing a QA program requires a commitment of time and resources. The design and scope of a QA program depends on the size and complexity of manufacturing practices performed by the establishment.

The technical, scientific, medical and administrative aspects of transfusion medicine continue to be critical. We all must find ways to provide a safer unit of blood and blood components.

However, there must be a realization by all involved in the profession that each of the above aspects deserves equal attention, respect and support. Why? It is very simple! without all aspects of transfusion medicine working together for the common good, the care of the patient, we will all fail.

References

1. Code of Federal Regulations, Title 21, Parts 200 to 299. "Food and Drugs". US Government Printing Office, Washington, DC, 1992.
2. Code of Federal Regulations, Title 21, parts 600 to 799. "Food and Drugs". US Government Printing Office, Washington, DC, 1992.
3. Quideline for Quality Assurance in Blood Establishments, (Docket No. 91N-0450). Food and Drug Administration, Rockville, Maryland, June 17, 1993.
4. Kotter J. A force for change: How leadership differs from management. The Free Press, A division of Macmillan, Inc., New York, NY, 1990.

BLOOD AND PLASMA PROCESSING: FACILITIES AND PHYSICAL REQUIREMENTS

S. Arnoldussen

Introduction

Products derived from human blood can be divided into two groups: Firstly, there are the products derived from single donations or small pools of source material (whole blood, cryoprecipitate, cell concentrates). These products are mainly unprocessed and are commonly used in transfusion medicine. The products from this group are covered by the EC Note for Guidance 111/8379/89-EN: "Medicinal products derived from human blood and plasma".

Secondly, there are products derived from human plasma and produced on an industrial scale from pools of source material. The products from this group are covered by the Directive 89/381/EEC, later included in the Directive 91/356/EEC. For both groups of products the principles of Good Manufacturing Practice (GMP) as laid down in Directive 91/356/EEC and the relevant "Guide to Good Manufacturing Practice for Medicinal Products" (The Rules Governing Medicinal Products in the EC, Volume IV) should be followed.

Regulatory authorities regard the site of manufacture of medicinal products derived from human blood or human plasma as an important factor determining the quality of the product. In Chapter 3 of the Guide to Good Manufacturing Practice for Medicinal Products (EC GMP Guide) the general requirements for premises in which manufacturing of medicinal products takes place, are laid down.

In principle, the main requirements for these premises are the following:

- They should be set up in a way which presents minimal risk for (cross)contamination of materials or products.
- They should allow for easy and effective cleaning.
- The environmental conditions in the facility should be such, that the quality of the product is not adversely affected.
- Steps should be taken to prevent unauthorized people from coming in.
- The premises should be designed and equipped so as to afford maximum protection against entry of insects or other animals.

This paper will focus on the implication of several requirements for premises used for the collection of blood and processing of blood products from single donations. The following items will be covered:

- Building design and layout of the facility: People flow, goods flow, restricted areas and segregation of activities.
- Construction and finishing: Materials to be used, finishing requirements.
- Environmental requirements: Room classification per type of activity, precautions concerning room classification (pressurisation, room entry, gowning procedures).

Building design and layout

The general requirements as laid down in the EC GMP Guide [1] are already mentioned above. In the introduction of Chapter 3 of these Guidelines it is stated that:

"Premises and equipment should be located, designed, adapted and maintained to suit the operations carried out.

Their layout should aim to minimize the risk of errors and to permit effective cleaning and maintenance in order to avoid cross-contamination, build up of dust or dirt, and, in general, any adverse effect on the quality of products."

Provisions of the EC GMP Guide [1], the 21 CFR 640.40 [2] and the WHO Requirements for Biological Substances No. 27, annex 4 [3] require that facilities for the collection and processing of blood and blood components shall:

- Provide adequate space for the following when applicable:
  - Private examination of donors
  - The withdrawal of blood from donors with minimal risk of contamination, or exposure to activities not related to blood collection
  - The storage of blood or blood components pending completion of tests
  - The quarantine storage of blood or blood components
  - The storage of finished products prior to distribution
  - The quarantine storage, handling and disposition of products and reagents not suitable for use
  - The orderly collection, processing, compatibility testing, storage and distribution of blood and blood components to prevent contamination
  - The adequate and proper performance of all steps of plasmapheresis, plateletapheresis and leukapheresis procedures
  - The orderly conduction of all packaging, labelling and other finishing operations
  - The storage of equipment
- Provide adequate lighting, ventilation and screening of open windows and doors.
- Provide adequate, clean and convenient handwashing facilities for personnel and adequate clean and convenient toilet facilities for donors and personnel. Drains shall be of adequate size, and, where connected directly to a sewer, shall be equipped with traps to prevent back-siphonage.
- Provide for safe and sanitary disposal for the following:

- Trash and items used during collection, processing and compatibility testing of blood and blood components
- Blood and blood components not suitable for distribution.

It is surprising that the FDA and WHO regulations more or less allow that laboratory activities be conducted in the same room as processing activities, although the FDA Plasmapheresis Inspection Instructions [4] state "a separate room for laboratory procedures is ideal, ...". EC GMPs require a separate testing laboratory [1], as well as the Dutch Guideline "Richtlijn GMP voor Bloedbanken" [5]. This last guideline is based primarily on the EC GMP Guidelines.

The above mentioned requirements imply that the routing of people and materials should be such, that the risk for errors and contamination are minimized. In practice this means that the facility should offer enough space to facilitate the work done and that activities are separated as much as possible. Provisions must be made to maintain a good hygiene (handwashing facilities, gowning areas) and a quarantine storage for non-released product and rejected materials should be available.

The facility preferably is set up such that the flow of process is followed, and crossing lines of product and material flows through the building are avoided.

The normal process flow through a blood collection center will be as follows: Blood collection, blood processing, laboratory activities, storage of product, packaging/labelling of products, storage, distribution and shipping.

The blood collection room

The room in which the collections take place should be a dedicated room, separate from other (processing) rooms. There should be a separate room for examinations [2,5], there should be enough space around the beds to facilitate the blood collection and all other activities necessary [3,6,7] and rooms should be available to receive and treat donors with adverse reactions [5].

The floors and walls should be made of material that is easy to clean and washable, and be installed without inaccessible corners and avoidance of internal window ledges [7]. Cleaning and disinfection is important if any contaminated blood is spilled. The rooms should have adequate ventilation and the temperature should be checked daily [7].

The processing area

This area should be separated from the rest of the facility, and should be dedicated to processing. The set up of the area should be such, that the flow of the process is followed and that production lines do not cross, in order to prevent mix-up of intermediates and products.

There should be sufficient space for temporary storage of intermediates. There should be no windows that can be opened [5]. The rooms should have adequate ventilation and the temperature should be checked daily [7].

The testing laboratory

Laboratories for testing and compatibility testing should be separate from the rest of the facility [1,5]. Laboratories should have separate gowning procedures as to avoid contamination and garments should be different from those worn in the processing facility. This implies a separate gowning room for the testing laboratory, or at least a separate route to follow for personnel entering the laboratory area.

Laboratories should have adequate ventilation and the temperature should be checked daily [7].

Storage areas

There are storage areas required for the following [2,5]:

- Quarantine storage in a separate room that can be locked.
- Separate storage of released product.
- Separate storage for rejected product, in an area that can be locked. Potentially infectious materials should be stored separately and must be removed from the facility as soon as possible.
- Storage of in-process materials.
- Separate storage of labels.

Storage areas should be of sufficient capacity to allow orderly storage of materials such as starting materials, packaging materials, intermediates and final product. Where special storage conditions are required (e.g. temperature) these should be checked and monitored.

Packaging area

As packaging materials as carton or unpainted wood are not allowed in the processing areas, packaging of finished products should take place in an area separate from the processing rooms. The packaging area does not necessarily have to be an area dedicated to packaging operations [6].

Distribution area

The distribution area should be located such that shipping of products can take place without passing the processing or other areas, in order to avoid a risk for mix-up of materials.

Ancillary areas

For the following auxiliary areas can be used:

- Gowning areas and handwashing facilities for processing, blood collection and for laboratory activities [4,5].
- A separate area for storage of cleaning materials [1].

Gowning up is a requirement when collecting and processing blood. Not only to protect the product, but to protect personnel as well. Gowning rooms should be available when entering each room where a different gowning procedure is required.

Disposal of contaminated waste

(Contaminated) waste from the processing area and the laboratory must be disposed of in a safe and sanitary manner [2]. If potentially infectious waste is not incinerated, then it should be sterilized for 60 min at 121°C [4].

It should be possible to dispose of contaminated waste from the laboratory without having to pass through the production area.

Entry to the facility

Persons whose presence can adversely affect the safety and purity of the products shall be excluded from areas where collection and processing of blood is conducted [2].

Unauthorized persons (such as donors) should not be able to enter the processing area.

The layout of the facility should be such, that personnel have to pass a controlled access gowning area or transfer area before entering the production facilities. Entry can be controlled, e.g. by identity cards.

Personnel should only be in those areas, where they have work to carry out.

Construction/Materials, finishing

The facilities for the collection and production of blood and blood components must permit effective cleaning. To facilitate cleaning, specific materials should be used to furbish walls, floors and ceiling in the following areas: Blood collection room, processing area, laboratory area and gowning rooms. Working surfaces should be smooth, impermeable, withstand disinfection and cleaning agents and not easily be damaged. Corners that are inaccessible, and windowledges should be avoided. Floors should be rounded up to the walls to avoid uncleanable recesses.

Walls, floors and ceiling in classified areas are often coated with a material that provides the necessary chemical resistance, smoothness and cleanability. The following materials can be used:

Vinyl sheets (e.g. Mipolam sheets)

Vinyl sheets are used to cover floors, and sometimes to cover walls. The advantage of these sheets is the possibility to apply them seamless, such that the interface between the wall and cove base is completely sealed off to provide a smooth, cleanable surface.

The disadvantage is that vinyl becomes slippery when wet, and that heavy mobile equipment will damage the vinyl cover.

Epoxy coating or polyurethane coating

Epoxy or polyurethane is poured on a concrete floor, and forms an impermeable, mechanically strong, coating.

Epoxy or polyurethane coating is more resistant to mechanical stress than polyvinyl sheets, but more difficult to apply.

Epoxy or polyurethane coating can be used to apply on walls.

Expoxy coated steel panels

Expoxy coated steel panels are often used for walls and ceiling in clean rooms. The panels are prefabricated, and are assembled in situ. Epoxy coated steel panels are smooth, but difficult to repair after damage, unless the whole panel is replaced.

Attention must be paid to the finishing of the seams between the panels. Epoxy coated steel panels are expensive, and cannot be used for floors.

Tiles

Tiles can be used to apply on walls. The use of tiles on floors is not recommended, because of the seams that are difficult to cover. Furthermore, with tiles it is impossible to form a coved base with the wall.

Spray coating of polyvinyl

Plaster walls can be coated with a spray coating of polyvinyl chloride; monolithic membrane applied in three layers (Cocoon or Tretoplast). The vinyl can be applied to completely seal the interface between the wall and cove base to provide a smooth, cleanable surface. This material seals off very well, but can easily be punctured by sharp objects.

Room classification and environmental quality

Blood collection room

Permanent blood collection areas should be ventilated by an airhandling system to avoid the need for open windows. Temperature and humidity control should be adequate to cope with the number of people likely to be in the room and with the heat output of equipment. A maximum/minimum thermometer should be installed and checked daily [7]. The above requirement is set to guarantee the comfort of donors and personnel, and to avoid entry of animals, such as insects, through open windows. No specific level of air-cleanliness is required [5].

In a normal room a three-fold air change rate and a recirculation rate of 85 per cent sufficient, depending on the total heat-load in the room and the cooling capacity of the system.

Processing areas

We distinguish processes that take place in a closed system, where no special environmental conditions are required, the processes where connections are made, for example between blood bags or equipment (here there is a small risk of contamination) and large scale manufacturing processes where product may be exposed to the environment.

Processes with a limited risk of microbial contamination

If there is a risk of contamination, a class D (class 100.000 Fed. St. 209D) environment is recommended [5]. Product exposed to the environment requires strict control of the air quality. The use of Laminar Flow Cabinets is recommended [7].

In order to reach a class D air grade, the EC GMP Guide states that the number of air change rates should be generally higher than 20, however, in practice an air change rate of 10 is sufficient to achieve grade D. The air should be filtered over High Efficiency Particulate Air (HEPA) filters [1]. For class D these do not necessarily have to be mounted in the ceiling, but can be placed in the main airducts of the air handling system.

If an airhandling system is used, GMPs require that the system is tested (validated) to prove that the system works according to the preset specifications. Furthermore, there should be a maintenance program to assure a good and troublefree operation of the system.

Large scale open processes

Open processes are likely those on an industrial scale and they fall into another category (aseptically manufactured sterile products) than the products made by the average blood collection center. For the manufacturing circumstances of these products Annex 1 (Manufacture of Sterile Medicinal Products) of the EC GMP Guide should be consulted. Discussing the requirements for aseptic manufacturing of medicinal products fall outside the scope of this paper.

References

1. The rules governing medicinal products in the EC, Volume IV: Guide to Good Manufacturing Practices for Medicinal Products. Commission of the European Communities. Office for official publications of the EC, Luxembourg, 1992. ISBN 92-826-3180-x.
2. Code of Federal Regulations title 21, part 606, subpart C. Food and Drug Administration. Office of the Federal Register, 1991.
3. WHO Technical Report Series, No 786, annex 4, 1989. WHO Expert Committee on Biological Standardization, World Health Organisation.
4. Plasmapheresis Inspection Checklist Instructions. Department of Health and Human Services, Food and Drug Administration. US Government Printing Office, 1990 261-215/24714.
5. Richtlijn GMP voor Bloedbanken. Blood Transfusion Council of the Netherlands Red Cross, september 1992.
6. Manufacture of products derived from human blood or human plasma, Annex to the EC Guide to GMP, III/3232/92-EN. Working Party on Control of Medicines and Inspections. Commission of the European Communities, Directorate-General Internal Market and Industrial Affairs, Brussels, 1993.
7. Guide to the preparation, use and quality assurance of blood components. Council of Europe Press, 1992. ISBN 92-871-1808-4.

DOCUMENTATION AND RECORD KEEPING: THE KEY TO COMPLIANCE

D.E. Nevalainen

Introduction

Good Manufacturing Practice (GMP) is described in one form or another in many countries for the purpose of guiding the manufacture, production and distribution of medical products and pharmaceuticals. The common theme contained in all of these documents is the description of what can best be called a system of documentation and records. The principles, hierarchy, and applications of such a documented quality system will be described.

Background

Good Manufacturing Practices (GMP) have come a long way since their introduction in the mid-sixties. GMP acceptance as a "way of life" has gradually become the norm in most developed countries. Spurred on by well publicized disasters and tragedy, regulatory authorities world wide have developed and adapted legally enforceable GMP codes [1]. The universal practices of GMP from the pharmaceutical environment [2,3] have gradually found their way into the blood bank environment [4-9] and are beginning to be broadly applied. The common theme running through all of these codified systems is that of *documentation and record keeping*. They all are various forms of a documentated quality system.

Such systems are characterized by four levels of hierarchy that have been described as 1) a Quality Manual, 2) System-level Procedures, 3) Work Instructions and 4) Records, Reports, and Forms [10]. An effective document system requires a systematic approach that covers all areas of an organization. The ISO 9000 approach to quality systems is one useful model [11-14] that is compatible with GMP. With the publication of the preproduction Quality Control (QC) guidelines in 1989 [15] the Food and Drug Administration (FDA) brought the US GMP regulations into line with the requirements of ISO 9001 [11].

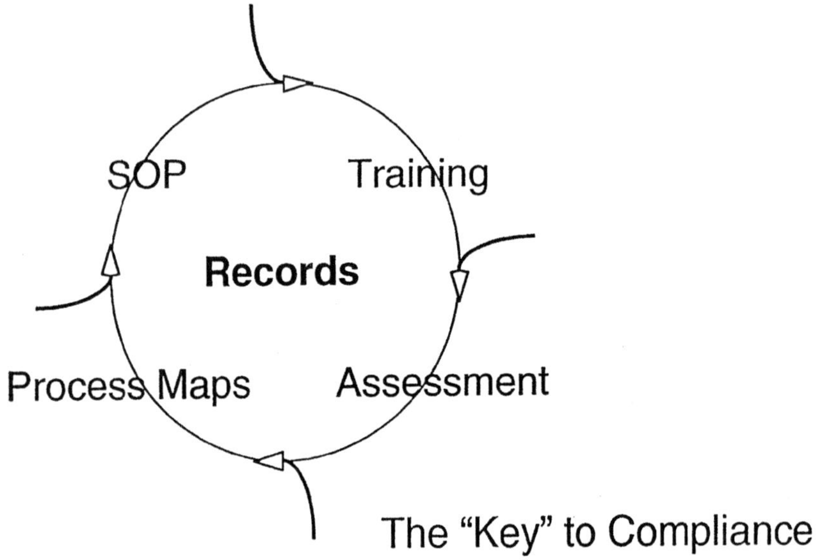

Figure 1. Elements of toal process control (GMP). Reprinted with permission of Abbott Quality Institute®.

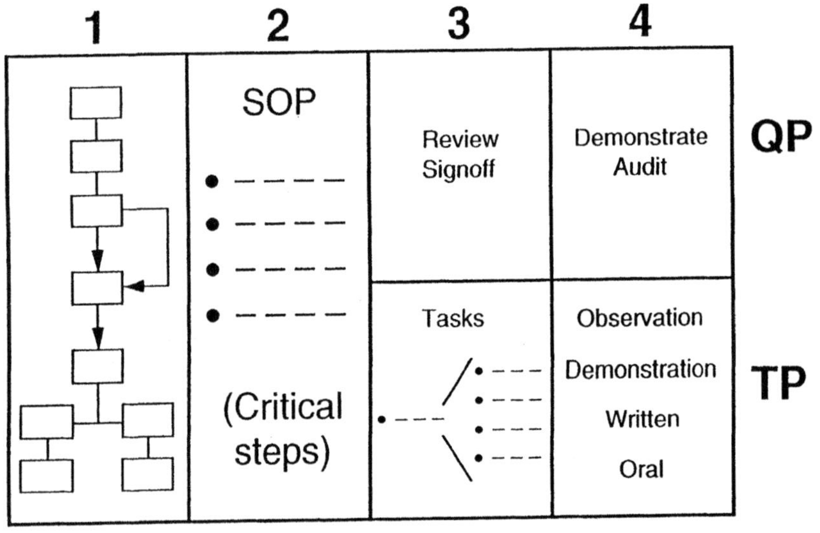

Figure 2. Pictorial representation of Process Mapping (1), Standard Operating Procedures (2), Training (3) and Assessment (4) from Figure 1. Reprinted with permission of Abbott Quality Institute®.

The quality system

Documents describe how the system should operate and may consist of guidelines for writing documents, change control documents, numbering systems, batch records, validation protocols, procedures, policies, work instructions, training procedures, and other documents necessary to support the activities of the organization. An overview of the five basic elements of a quality system is seen in Figure 1. The document development and implementation characteristics are seen on the outer circle. Records are the core process that creates the audit trail used to demonstrate that the documents are being used properly to meet system requirements. The arrows on the periphery represent entry points where people will interact with the existing documents, or will provide a template map for document development and/or change. You will notice that there is no start or stop point in the circle. The quality journey never stops, and improvements should be ongoing at all times [16]. Document development is the basic process upon which the entire system depends. Without a good, user friendly document which is trainable, the system will not work consistently. Figure 2 is a schematic representation of the elements listed on the circle.

The process begins with process mapping (flow charting) to identify the critical steps or stages of a process (step 1). The process map serves as a template for the Standard Operating Procedure (SOP) which will list the critical steps and provide additional information regarding purpose, scope, etc. (step 2). Quality Procedures (QP) and Technical Procedures (TP) require different degrees of detail for the third step of the process, the training documents. For TP each critical step can be broken up into its constituent tasks and/or competencies and described in as much detail as necessary, while QP may need only a review and signature. Step 4 is the competency assessment process which can be used to certify employees for a specific SOP [17-20]. Examples of a process map, an SOP, a training document, and an assessment form is found as attachments 1 and 2. Attachement 3 is a sample certification form which can be used to document that all requirements for certification are in place (records). The key to writing good documents is to keep them simple, clear, and concise, with lots of "white space". Put all the detail (the black stuff) in an associated training document. Since the SOP is a "regulated" document, every time it gets touched a record is required. One can make minor changes to the training document without changing the SOP. This structure simplifies the document management process.

The work process

Any information, or material that is turned into products or services must go through some process that adds value to it in such a way as to make someone wish to purchase the product or service. The GMP process can be viewed in this same way (Figure 3). The work process within any organization is a unique blend of methods, people, machines, and environment, coupled with measurements in key places. The document system describes how the system should

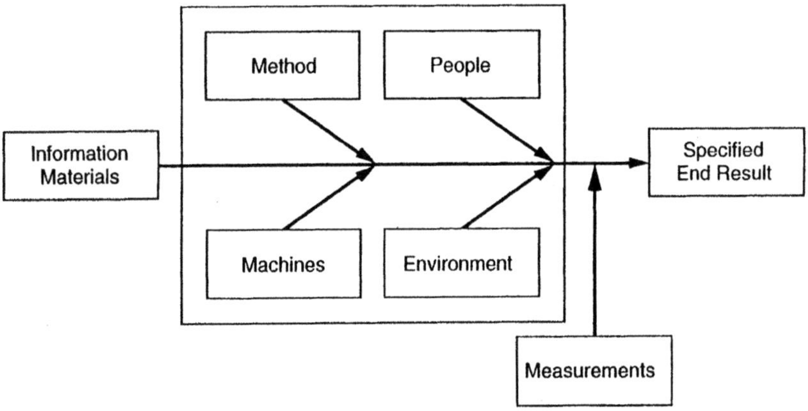

Figure 3. Process overview. Reprinted with permission of Abbott Quality Institute®.

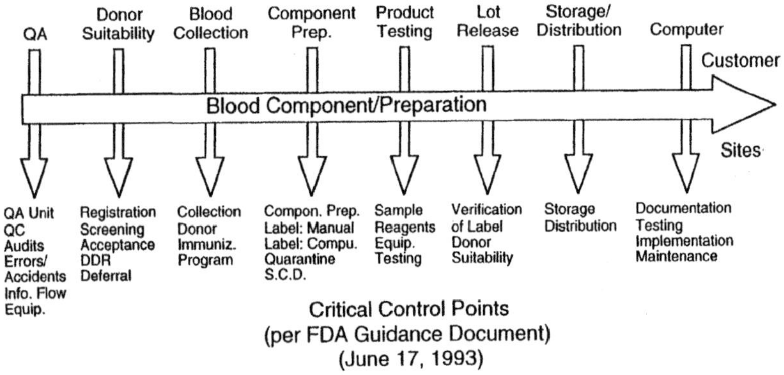

Figure 4. Blood Bank system. Reprinted with permission of Abbott Quality Institute®.

operate, and records provide the audit trail to ensure that the system is operating according to system specifications [19,20]. Because no two organizations are identical, the document and recordkeeping system must be uniquely adapted to the system requirements.

In the Quality Assurance Guidance Document issued by the FDA [9] eight critical control points are described. The eight control points have been rearranged and spread out on a product preparation time-line (Figure 4). Each of these control points represents a process that is part of the larger blood bank system. This grid provides an overview of the types of documents, forms and records that may need to be considered for each area. Each critical control point is further broken down into subunits in the original document to provide a more detailed perspective to system specifications.

In considering what documents and records are necessary, one should be sure to direct the documents to the actual work process, not to the way people are organized. Figure 5 shows that people are organized in vertical arrays, while the actual work process of a blood bank is organized in a horizontal direction. It is important to analyze the work process to ensure that only those documents that are required are developed. Developing document systems around people will many times produce documents and work activities that may not be optimized to the work process, thereby contributing to variable output. Figure 6 shows how a process can be broken down to subprocesses, activities, and even to specific tasks. Documents should describe how each of these functions inter-relate to each other, and form the operating specifications for the system. Again, the records will be the basis of the audit trail that demonstrates that the system is working to its specifications. A GMP system is characterized by the terms Documentation, Training and Tracking (traceability) [19]. Process improvements using flowcharting techniques and the seven tools statistical process control [21] can have an impact by decreasing the numbers of steps in a process, thereby reducing the numbers of documents required in the system as was demonstrated at in a case study at LDS Hospital Blood Bank in Salt Lake city Utah [22].

Software/Computer considerations

As the regulatory authorities increase their enforcement activities, many regulated companies are finding it necessary to improve their GMP compliance programs. In order to improve both compliance and productivity, many companies are turning to commercially available manufacturing software. In the past several years, the number of off the shelf manufacturing software packages designed for GMP regulated companies has increased. Such packages are available to track calibration of measurement equipment, product stability, customer complaints, and GMP training activities. In analyzing the recordkeeping needs for a GMP application, the user should pay attention to two types of information: A description of the amount and types of data to be tracked and stored, and a step by step flow of the data. A system that tracks the calibration of measurement equipment, for example, might describe the calibration due date as a date field in the format

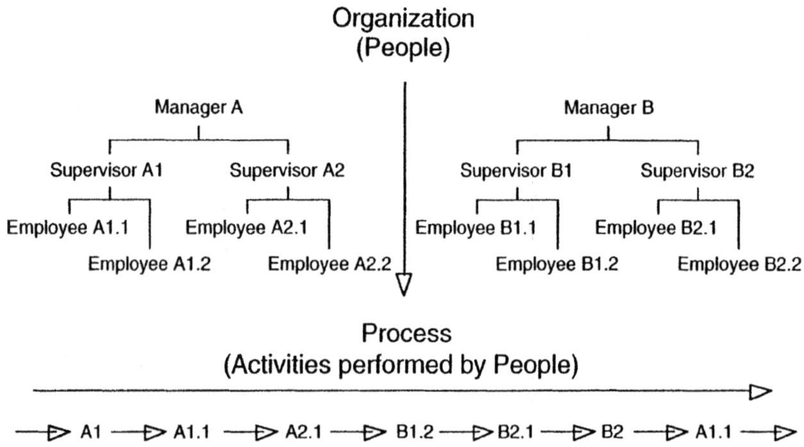

Figure 5. Organizations vs. Process. Reprinted with permission of Abbott Quality Institute®

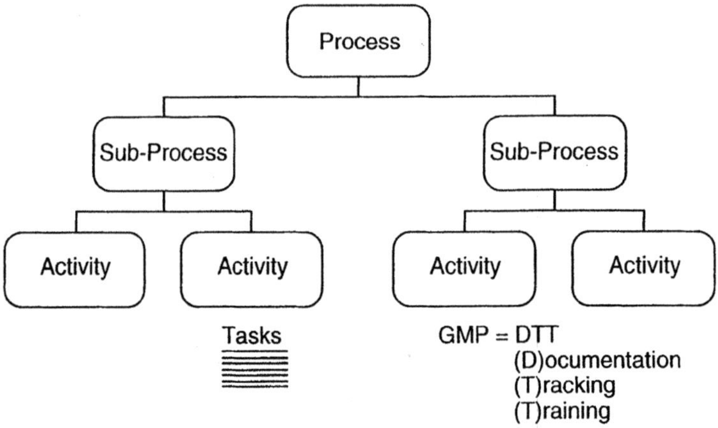

Figure 6. The Process Concept. Reprinted with permission of Abbott Quality Institute®.

month/day/year. A description of the data flow should include how the data are to be stored and manipulated. A simplified description of data flow for a calibration system may include what items are due to be calibrated, printing the calibration forms, calibrating the items, entering the calibration records, and calculating new calibration dates. A flow chart is useful in this context because it provides a concise way to present complex information [23]. Regulatory recordkeeping standards demand consistency, accuracy, traceability, accountability, and reliability. The best GMP software will be designed to achieve these requirements. Specific features that will ensure the integrity of the data include:

- *Audit trail:* A method of showing the history of all changes to a given record.
- *Access control:* Usually a password system to ensure that only authorized personnel have access to the system.
- *Data entry validation:* A method for minimizing the entry of incorrect or invalid data.
- *Data archive:* A separate data base where inactive records can be stored for easy retrieval.
- *Data backup:* A means to make a duplicate set of data which can be reinstalled should there be a problem with the original.
- *Record deletion protection:* A method to eliminate the accidental or malicious deletion of records, usually accomplished by access control and built-in safeguards [23].

GMP documentation requirements for automated systems have been well described by Tetzlaff [24]. Computers, like any other equipment or apparatus used in manufacturing or control operations, must be demonstrably functioning a proper manner. Several sections of the CFR (US FDA) are relevant to computers used for GMP functions and include but are not limited to: Part 211.68 Automatic, mechanical, and electronic equipment, part 211.160 Laboratory controls, general requirements, part 211.165 Testing and release for distribution, and part 211.194 which states that the "suitability of all testing methods shall be verified under actual conditions of use". If computer checks are performed in a scientifically sound manner, it is unlikely that investigators will find faults. Unfortunately inspections continue to find instances in which computer systems have not been adequately validated, or have not been validated at all [24]. One of the eight critical control points described in the FDA Quality Assurance (QA) guideline [9] is focused on computer systems and presents a rational overview of the necessary elements of for documentation of computer related systems. Implementing a computer documentation system requires a great deal of thought and planning. An efficient computer documentation system will pay for itself through time savings and improved access to vital information. It is important that all features of the system be documented to enable appropriate validation to be performed [25].

Summary

Applying general pharmaceutical GMP practice patterns to the "blood bank industry" continues to be debated in many circles [26,27]. Despite the debate, when GMP is viewed as a quality system, the process controls required by GMP are useful and valid approaches to the management of complex processes, and more importantly, allows one to have control over them. It is helpful to think of GMP as a quality system. When reviewing the list of common deficiencies in ISO 9000 quality system assessment audits regarding documents one sees repeatedly such things as a) unapproved documents in use, b) procedures don't match practices (failure to follow SOP), c) unofficial changes in the procedure, d) obsolete documentation in use, and e) documents are not located where they are supposed to be. Common people related deficiencies include a) not trained or otherwise qualified for their jobs, b) not aware of requirements, c) don't have access to procedures, d) not complying with procedures, e) organization and responsibilities not as described in quality manual, and f) temporary employees not included in the system [10]. Those deficiencies sound very similar to the FDA 483 citations coming from the Blood Bank Inspection process as published by the "*citings information exchange*" [28]. Using the ISO 9000 or quality systems approach may make it easier to understand the quality reasons for setting up a proper document and recordkeeping system. Surprisingly enough, when done this way ... GMP just happens!

References

1. Sharp J. Good manufacturing practice: Philosophy and application. Buffalo Grove, Interpharm Press, 1991.
2. Food and Drug Administration. Code of Federal Regulations. 21 CFR Parts 210-211 Pharmaceutical GMP, USA.
3. Commission of the European Communities. Rules for governing medicinal products in the European Community. Volume IV. Good manufacturing practice for medicinal products. Luxembourg, 1992.
4. College voor de Bloedtransfusie. Richtlijn GMP voor bloedbanken. Amsterdam, College voor de Bloedtransfusie van het Nederlandse Rode Kruis, 1992.
5. United Kingdom Blood Transfusion Service/National Institute for Biological Standards and Control. Guidelines for the blood transfusion services in the United Kingdom, 1989.
6. Loeber JG, Slagter S. Code of practice for implementation of a quality system in laboratories in the health care sector. 1st ed. CCKL Bilthoven, The Netherlands, 1991.
7. World Health Organization, Expert Committee of Biological Standardization. Requirements for the collection, processing, and quality control of blood, blood components, and plasma derivatives. Geneva, 1991.
8. Food and Drug Administration. Code of Federal Regulations. 21 CFR Part 606 GMP for Blood and Blood Components, USA.
9. Food and Drug Association, Center for Biologics Evaluation and Research. Guideline for quality assurance in blood establishments. June 17, 1993.
10. Stat-A-Matrix Institute. ISO 9000 awareness program. Edison: Stat-A-Matrix Institute, 1993.

11. American National Standards Institute/American Society for Quality Control. Q91: Quality systems-model for quality assurance in design/development, production, installation and servicing. Milwaukee, ASQC, 1987.
12. Henke C. ISO 9000: Choice or necessity? Med Dev Diag Ind 1992;Oct:44-48,86-88.
13. Byrnes D. Exploring the world of ISO 9000. Quality 1992;Oct:19-31.
14. Bureau of Business Practice. ISO 9000: Handbook of quality standards and compliance. 1992.
15. Food and Drug Administration, Center for Devices and Radiological Health. Preproduction quality assurance planning: Recommendations for medical device manufacturers. September 1989.
16. Imai M. Kaizen. The key to Japan's competitive succes. 1st ed. McGraw Hill, New York, 1986.
17. Nevalainen DE. Laboratory apprenticeships: A lookback in history or a new paradigm? Clin Lab Man Rev 1993;580:573-7.
18. Nevalainen DE, Berte LM. Training, verification, and assessment: Keys to quality management. Clinical Laboratory Management Association, 1993.
19. Nevalainen DE. Total process control in the blood bank and laboratory environment: Process analysis and management. Abbott Quality Institute, Chicago, 1993.
20. Nevalainen DE. Total process control in the blood bank and laboratory environment: Principles and philosophy of good manufacturing practice. Abbott Quality Institute, Chicago, 1993.
21. Brassard M. The memory jogger: A pocket guide of tools for continuous improvement. Methuen, GOAL/QPC, 1988.
22. Beesley J, Helton HD, Merkley A, Swalberg ED. How we implemented TQM in our laboratory and blood bank. Clin Lab Man Rev 1993;Jan:219-27.
23. Erickson JR. Selecting software for GMP applications. Med Dev Diag Ind 1993;Jan:122-8.
24. Tetzlaff RF. GMP documentation requirements for automated systems. Part III. FDA inspections of computerized laboratory systems. Pharm Tech 1992;May:70-83.
25. Carr J, Eddy M, Rego A. On-line documentation. Med Dev Diag Ind 1993;Feb:53-60.
26. Menitove JE. Controversies in transfusion medicine. The recent emphasis on good manufacturing practices and the pharmaceutical manufacturing approach damages blood banking and transfusion medicine as medical care activities: Con. Transfusion 1993;33:439-42.
27. Miller MV. Controversies in transfusion medicine. Blood banks should use good manufacturing practices and the pharmaceutical manufacturing approach: Pro. Transfusion 1993;33:435-8.
28. Citings Information Exchange. 1899-B Billingsgate Circle, Richmond VA 23233, USA.

Attachement 1

Process Analysis: ***Appendix F ... Sample Procedure and Training***

MCRIT.ACL 2a1
DONOR ROOM SPUN MICROHEMATORICT Page: 1

```
Fill Two cap.tubes (1/2 to 2/3 full).
Seal One end of each with Clay.
Load into Centrifuge.
Set Timer for Five Minutes.
Read the results.
Interpret and record the results:
    (Allogeneic Donor) Is the hematocrit 38% or greater?
        (Yes) Accept the donor.
        (No)  Temporarily defer the donor per SP XXXX.
    ?end
    (Autologous donor) Is the hematocrit 33% or greater?
        (Yes) Accept the donor.
        (No)  Temporarily defer the donor per SP XXXX.
    ?end
:end
```

DRAFT — Process Analysis and Management
September 20, 1993 — Abbott Quality Institute®, Diagnostics Division, Abbott Laboratories

Process Analysis: ***Appendix F ... Sample Procedure and Training***

2b1
Page: 1

MCRIT2.ACL
μHEMATOCRIT PROCEDURE SP.0101OPA ——— ***Proc. Document Number***
{David E. Nevalainen 01 SEP 93} ——— ***Author and Date***

```
{01} Fill Two cap.tubes (1/2 to 2/3 full).
{02} Seal One end of each with Clay.
{03} Load into Centrifuge.
{04} Set Timer for Five Minutes.
{05} Read the results.
{06} Interpret and record the results:
         (Allogeneic Donor) Is the hematocrit 38% or greater?
             (Yes) Accept the donor.
             (No)  Temporarily defer the donor per SP XXXX.
         ?end
         (Autologous donor) Is the hematocrit 33% or greater?
             (Yes) Accept the donor.
             (No)  Temporarily defer the donor per SP XXXX.
         ?end
     :end
```

Steps in SOP

DRAFT — Process Analysis and Management
September 20, 1993 — Abbott Quality Institute®, Diagnostics Division, Abbott Laboratories

μHEMATOCRIT PROCEDURE SP.0101OPA

Proc. Document # 2c1

ABBOTT QUALITY INSTITUTE
System Procedure Manual
Section Name: *Collections*

System Procedure #: SP0101.OPA
Page #: 1 of 2
Date : 01 SEP 93

SYSTEM PROCEDURE COVER PAGE

SP0101.OPA **Microhematocrit (Donor)**

DISTRIBUTION	DEPT.: 01 – COLLECTIONS	COPIES: 1 – 6
	DEPT.: 04 – QUALITY ASSURANCE	COPIES: 7
	DEPT.: 05 – REGULATORY	COPIES: 8
	DEPT.: ______________	COPIES:
	______________	COPIES:
	______________	COPIES:
	______________	COPIES:

ISSUED BY: DEPT.: QUALITY ASSURANCE

WRITTEN BY: DEPT.: COLLECTIONS (01)

REV. #	DATE	DESCRIPTION	REASON	SIGN-OFF	DOCUMENT CTRL DATE	DOCUMENT CTRL SIGN
A	01SEP93	Individual Draft				

ABBOTT QUALITY INSTITUTE	System Procedure # : SP0101.OPA
System Procedure Manual	Page # : 2/3 of 3
Section Name: *Collections*	Date : 01 SEP 93

SYSTEM PROCEDURE

SP0101.OPA **Microhematocrit (Donor)**

1.0 **PURPOSE**

The purpose of this procedure is to describe the method for performing the microhematocrit procedure on donors to determine whether they should be deferred for low hemoglobin levels.

2.0 **SCOPE**

This procedure is for use in the donor selection process, in both fixed and mobile collection sites.

3.0 **PROCEDURE**

Equipment Required: Microhematocrit Centrifuge; Heparinized Capillary tubes; Sealing clay; Microhematocrit reader

Responsible Personnel

Donor Room Nures

NOTE: These steps correlate with steps in MCRIT2.ACL process flow.

3.01	Fill two (2) capillary tubes 1/2 to 2/3 full from a free flowing finger stick or ear lobe punture.
3.02	Seal one end of each tube with clay.
3.03	Place into centrifuge.
3.04	Set timer for five (5) minutes.
	Read and record results.
3.06	Interpret results.

4.0 **REFERENCES**

4.01 J.B. Henry. Clinical Diagnosis And Management By Laboratory Methods. 18th Ed. W.B. Saunders, 1991, pgs. 560-561.

5.0 **DEFINITIONS**

5.01 *Hematocrit* – packed red cell volume in donor's blood.

5.02 *Deferral* – rejection of donor due to a hematocrit below a predetermined level.

5.03 *Autologous* – blood collected and stored for transfusion into the donor (self) at a point of time in the future. (A recipient receives his/her own blood back in a routine transfusion procedure).

5.04 *Allogeneic* – a regular blood donation that is intended for use in recipients other than the donor – not autologous (see above).

6.0 **RECORDS**

6.01 Donor History Card with records of present donation.

6.02 Hematocrit procedure log sheet.

7.0 **ATTACHEMENTS OR APPENDICES**

7.01 Sample donor history record.

7.02 Sample laboratory log sheet for hematocrit procedure.

7.03 Process map for microhematocrit procedure.

Doc. # (Training Guide) 2d1/2

ABBOTT QUALITY INSTITUTE	System Procedure # :	SP0101.TRN
System Procedure Manual	Page # :	1/2 of 2
Section Name: *Collections*	Revised :	01 SEP 93

SYSTEM PROCEDURE TRAINING GUIDE

TASKS / CRITERIA / ASSESSMENT

REFERENCE PROCEDURE: SP0101.OPA Microhematocrit (Donor)

TRAINING METHODS:

Using tube of anti-coagulated blood:

1. Observe process
2. Practice process under supervision
3. Demonstrate successful hematocrit procedure

Pass oral quiz on procedure and process.

PROCEDURAL STEPS:

3.01 Fill capillary tubes by gravity.
Free-flowing puncture.
No clots.

3.02 Sealrite or equivalent.
1/8 to 1/4 inch of clay needed.
Push straight in to prevent breakage and potential injury.

3.03 Place into centrifuge with clay to the outside. Place tubes opposite each other.
Record slot numbers if more than one donor is being spun simultaneously.
Screw down protective cover.
Put lid down and snap latch.

3.04 Set timer for five (5) minutes to obtain maximum packing of blood cells. Less time will give a falsely elevated hematocrit.

3.05 Use standard hematocrit reader provided to obtain percentage packed cells. (equipment # XXXXX).
Dispose of capillary tubes in appropriate waste container for sharps. (Biohazardous).
Record the hematocrit result on the appropriate donor history form and the hematocrit log sheet.

These steps correlate with steps in SOP.

3.06 Interpretation:

Allogeneic (Regular) Donor: If the hematocrit is 38% or greater the donor meets the minimum requirement and may proceed to the next step. If the hematocrit is less than 38% the donor should be temporarily deferred per System Procedure XXXX.

Autologous Donor: If the hematocrit is 33 % or greater the donor meets the minimum requirement and may proceed to the next step. If the hematocrit is less than 33% the donor should be temporarily deferred per System Procedure XXX.

4.0 **REFERENCES**

4.01 J.B. Henry. Clinical diagnosis and management by laboratory methods. 18th ed. W.B. Saunders, 1991, pgs. 560-561.

4.02 Technical Manual. 11th edition. American Association of Blood Banks. Bethesda, MD, 1993, p. 12.

4.03 Operations Manual for IEC Centrifuge No. XXXX.

4.04 Microhematocrit procedure SP0101.OPA (Attached)

4.05 Microhematocrit Process Map SP0101.PMA (Attached)

4.06 Oral and written examination questions and answers (Attached)

Attachment 2
Job Training and Certification: ***Appendix E ... Job Competency analysis***

page 1 of 1 *Abbbott Quality Institute®*
********SAMPLE ONLY********

Edition No. ____________________
Document No. ____________________
Effective Date: ____________________

ABC CORPORATION, Inc.
(Department Name)
Job Competency Analysis For Job Certification
(Job Title)

Trainee's Signature/Employee No.: ____________________

Date: ____________ FOR INCOMING PLASMA ONLY YES/NO STP: ____________________

This JOB COMPETENCY ANALYSIS is meant to be performed at the work-site where an actual or simulated qualitative assay is being performed. You are to record whether the proper procedures, methods, and documents are used in order to perform the assay and if the assay is satisfactorily or unsatisfactorily performed.

DID THE RETROVIRUS/HEPATITIS TECHNICIAN PROPERLY:	YES	NO
1. Assemble all of the necessary materials needed to start the assay?		
2. Use pipets/laboratory equipment?		
3. Take all appropriate safety measures?		
4. Perform the testing in accordance with area OPs, EOPs, Guidelines, Policies, STPs and SCPs?		
5. Use proper aseptic technique?		
6. Evaluate results and interpret data?		
8. Complete all paperwork?		
9. Perform all HP/AMM transactions?		

ADDITIONAL NOTES/COMMENTS: ____________________

Note: These comments will become part of trainee's permanent file.

Evaluator's Signature: ____________________
Date/Time of Evaluation: ____________________

Attachment 3
Job Training and Certification: ***Appendix D ... Training Outline for Job Certifications***

page 1 of 4

Edition No. ____________________ Effective Date: ________________

ABC CORPORATION, Inc.
(Department Name)
Job Outline For Job Certification
(Area Title)

Employee's Name: ______________________ Employee Number: ____________
Employee SSN: ____________

Start Date: ________Date In Job: _____ _____ Date Completed: ____________
Supervisor's Name: ____________________ Dept. Number: ____________

Trainer's Name/Signature ____

		Date Completed
I.	Organization Knowledge	
	a. Orientation	________________
	b. Process Overview	________________
	d. Terminology (if unique)	________________
	d. Facility Tour	________________
	e. Safety Training	________________
II.	Departmental Knowledge	
	a. Area Tour	________________
	b. Dress Requirements	________________
	c. Department Terminology	________________
	d. General Rules and Regulations	________________
III.	Quality Knowledge	
	a. Good Manufacturing Practice	________________
	b. Understanding the Quality Organization	________________
	c. Labels/Labelling GMP	________________

Document Number: ____________________

Abbbott Quality Institute®
*******SAMPLE ONLY*******

Edition No. ______________________

ABC CORPORATION, Inc.

(Department Name)

Job Outline For Job Certification

(Area Title)

IV. General Job Related ______________ ______________

1st Review 2nd Review

1. Document Number 1 and its Title/Name
   Policy.xx.

2. Document Number 2 and its Title/Name
   Policy.xx.

3. ETC>

Examples from Abbott Laboratories:

1. Lot Number Assignment Using the xxxxx Software OP.A100
2 Document Signatures and Entries OP.A250
3. Biohazardous Spill Cleanup OP.C111
4. Solid Biohazardous, Non-radioactive and Solid Bioharzardous Radioactive Waste Disposal for the Qualitative AQA Laboratory OP.C105
5. General Instructions for Work with Human Serum or Plasma OP.C171
6. Housekeeping Procedures, AP8B 2nd Floor OP.D123

ETC>

Abbbott Quality Institute®

*******SAMPLE ONLY*******

page 3 /4of 4

Edition No. ____________________

ABC CORPORATION, Inc.

(Department Name)

Job Outline For Job Certification

(Area Title)

V. General Job Related ____________________ ____________________

1st Review 2nd Review

1. Document Number 1 and its Title/Name
   Policy.xx.
2. Document Number 2 and its Title/Name
   Policy.xx.
3. ETC>

Examples from Abbott Laboratories:

1. Maintenance of Temperature Records for Controlled Temperature Units OP.E101
2 Calibration of Dispensing Devices, AQA Qualitative Laboratory OP.E108
3. Operations and Maintenance of a Quantum II OP.E112
4. User Standardization of Timing Devices OP.E293
5. Product Stability Testing OP.L352
6. Setup, Standardization, Use of pH Meters EOP.EP102
7. Respiratory Protection: Selection and Use OP.A103
8. ETC>

VI. General Job Related ____________________ ____________________

Completion Date Authorized By

a. Procedure/Policy/Guideline Review ____________________
b. GMP/Quality Review ____________________
c. Job Competency Analysis ____________________
d. Evaluation ____________________
e. Defect Recognition (if applicable) ____________________

Abbbott Quality Institute®

*******SAMPLE ONLY*******

VALIDATION PROCEDURES AND INTERNAL AUDIT SYSTEMS

B. Cuthbertson

Introduction

Recent European legislation has brought some aspects of transfusion practice under regulatory control, particularly with regard to the collection of plasma for fractionation. For example, EEC Directive 89/381 extended the scope of previous directives to include special provisions for medicinal products derived from human blood or human plasma. Although this Directive does not apply to whole blood or other single donor products, Directive 91/507 requires manufacturers of licensed blood products to certify the quality of donor plasma. Finally, an Ad Hoc EEC Working Party issued a note for guidance covering medicinal products derived from human blood or plasma [1]. This document requires that each transfusion center should establish, document and maintain an effective Quality Assurance (QA) system.

Any effective QA system will have many components, which must be developed and maintained. In this presentation validation and audit will be discussed, because these are clearly key aspects of any quality system. Many of the other components of a quality system are discussed elsewhere in these proceedings.

Validation

The definition of validation given in the EEC Guide to Good Manufacturing Practices (GMP) [2] is as follows:

"Action of proving, in accordance with the principles of Good Manufacturing Practice, that any procedure, process, equipment, material, activity or system actually leads to the expected results."

This is a good definition which emphasizes the need to carry out some form of validation of almost all activities carried out in any pharmaceutical organization, including plasma fractionators and transfusion centers. Many of the requirements for validation and the required specifications are published elsewhere [2-6]. This section of the presentation will attempt to highlight the key issues which are required to be addressed in implementing an effective validation program.

Documentation of validation

Documentation is absolutely crucial to the success of any validation program. Indeed, it should be emphasized that if there is no documentary record of a validation exercise, then it cannot be considered that any validation was done at all.

All validation must be planned properly in advance and a detailed written test protocol should be generated before any validation work is started. This protocol should include details of the test methods to be used and the acceptability criteria (i.e. test limits). Once the validation has been carried out, it is important that a final report is generated which will include:
- Agreed validation protocol.
- Results of validation studies.
- Demonstration of conformance with acceptability criteria.
- Conclusions.
- Approval.

The extent of the work required to complete the validation will depend on the nature and complexity of the product or process being assessed. Thus, the size of the validation report may vary from a single page to a very substantial dossier.

The final approval will normally be given by a nominated member of the QA department. The validation report must then be filed carefully and retained for inspection by any relevant person, especially regulatory bodies. From personal experience at the Protein Fractionation Center it has frequently been found that validation reports have been referred to many times and are treated as key sources of data which are archived indefinitely.

Responsibility for validation

Validation is an integral part of any organization's quality system and as such is the responsibility of many sections of the organization. Validation need not be carried out within the organization, but in all cases the organization's QA department must ensure that it is carried out properly and documented properly. The QA department must also ensure that it is carried out at the correct times and to the correct specifications.

Types of validation

There are several different types of validation which must be carried out at different times. These types of validation will be illustrated by examples taken from standard transfusion practice. This should, hopefully, illustrate that much routine practice, which is taken for granted, can be considered as validation and complies with the definition of validation given earlier.

Pre-commissioning validation

The introduction of new manufacturing processes, new equipment, new assay methods or new premises must be controlled extremely carefully. Any such new activity must be validated fully and documented before it is introduced into routine use. Each organization should develop an effective system for reviewing all such new developments before they are approved for use. In addition, it is also essential that the commissioning program includes documentation (SOPs, etc.) which should be tested for accuracy during the validation procedure. A few examples will illustrate the meaning of pre-commissioning validation.

– *New manufacturing methods* must be validated before they are used to generate clinical products. For example, any new system for manufacturing platelet concentrate would have to be validated to demonstrate that the resultant product met or bettered the existing quality criteria and stability criteria, before the concentrate was used clinically. It is essential that this type of validation is carried out within the transfusion center, because a key aspect of the validation is to demonstrate that the method can be carried out reliably by the local staff who will implement it routinely.

– *New assay methods* also require validation before they are introduced for routine donation testing. This is especially important for test kits for donor testing for virological markers such as HBsAg, anti-HCV and anti-HIV. In the US, kit validation is partly the responsibility of the FDA, who license test kits for routine use. In Europe, there is no body which licenses test kits and, it is the responsibility of the user to ensure that any test used is fully validated before it is used for routine donation testing. In Scotland, no test kit may be used unless it has been validated in a multi-centered evaluation which includes the following:

- A test for specificity, by testing at least 5,000 donations.
- A test for sensitivity, using a panel of samples generated by an expert laboratory, to include dilutions of known positive samples, seroconversion samples and international standards where available (e.g. HBsAg).
- Validation of any test equipment (diluters, spectrophotometers, computer programs, etc.)

Again, it is crucial that staff gain hands on experience of any new test before it can be considered validated for routine testing.

– *New equipment* such as plasmapheresis machines and automated virology testing systems also require pre-commissioning validation. An essential component of equipment validation is to confirm that any operating software is fully tested for accuracy. It is not acceptable to assume that the manufacturer has not made any errors in programming the equipment and that it will automatically perform to the user specification. It is, of course, perfectly acceptable that the validation of new equipment is partly carried out by the equipment manufacturer, provided that a written validation and commissioning report is received from the manufacturer.

– *New premises* also require pre-commissioning validation to confirm that the design criteria have been met. This is especially important for all controlled environments, such as cold rooms and clean rooms, where it is essential to demonstrate that the correct specification is achieved.

For example, the European Pharmacopoeia are about to publish a specification for plasma for fractionation which requires that it is stored at a temperature below -30°C. Any new cold store must be subjected to temperature mapping

Table 1. Some suggestions for part of a validation programme.

Area	Equipment	Type of validation required	Suggested frequency
Processing	Centrifuges	Temperature control Rotor speed Times	3 monthly
	Laminar flow cabinets	Air flow HEPA filters	3-6 monthly
	Blast freezer	Temperature control Freezing rate	3 monthly
	All temperature controlled equipment	Check calibration of temperature recorders Check temperature	3 monthly
	Balances	Weight check	Daily
Virology	Sample handling equipment	Carryover Sample taking Accuracy of dilution	6 monthly
	Incubators	Check temperature	3 monthly
	Washers	Wash volume delivery	3 monthly
	Readers	OD standard check for each channel	Daily
	Reporting	Manually check print outs from reader	3 monthly

Table 2. Example of a validation programme for autoclaves.

1. Pre-commissioning	Full temperature mapping of chamber Temperature mapping of all loads, container types, etc. Calibration of recorders, probes, etc. Full validation report
2. Routine validation	
2.1 Every run	Check recording
2.2 Regular periods (e.g. quarterly)	Routine maintenance Recalibration of recorders, probe, etc. Temperature mapping of chamber

over a period of several days in order to demonstrate that this specification is complied with. The temperature recording equipment supplied with the cold store should be carefully calibrated against an independently certified temperature measuring system.

Routine validation of key equipment

Once equipment has been commissioned and is in routine use, it is essential that it is maintained in the correct operational condition. For some equipment, this will require regular maintenance by trained engineers. When such maintenance takes place, it is normally necessary to re-validate the equipment. Other items of equipment will not require regular maintenance, but will still require regular routine re-validation. A detailed validation program should be drawn up which gives details of the type of validation and frequency required for each key item of equipment. Recommendations for a validation program have been published by the Council of Europe [4]. Further suggestions for a validation program for equipment used in a transfusion center were drawn up by a working party within the SNBTS. These suggestions are given in Table 1. A further, more detailed, example covering the validation of an autoclave is given in Table 2. This type of routine validation requires a detailed validation schedule which should be monitored regularly for compliance.

Routine validation of performance

All routine manufacturing methods and laboratory assays must be validated routinely to confirm that performance remains within agreed specifications. This type of validation applies to a range of routine measurements, e.g.

- Markers of product quality.
- Product sterility.
- Assay control measurements.
- Product yield.

All such data should be collected against a defined program. It is essential that data is collated and reviewed on a regular basis. It is also suggested that the data is analyzed using a suitable statistical method, such as one or other form of statistical process control [7], in order to demonstrate any underlying trends in performance.

Validation of microbiological quality

A further component of an integrated validation program is the performance of routine microbiological monitoring of the manufacturing environment. A typical microbiological validation program would include:

- Air sampling of key manufacturing areas.
- Swab samples taken of centrifuge bowls and product storage areas.
- Contact (Rodac) plates taken of critical surfaces e.g. laminar flow cabinets.
- Validation of the effectiveness of disinfectants.

Such data should also be collated and reviewed regularly to confirm compliance with written specifications.

Auditing for GMP compliance

Requirement for audit

The requirement for GMP auditing is clearly stated in the EEC Guide to GMP [2] which includes the following statement:

"The system of Quality Assurance appropriate for the manufacture of medicinal products should ensure that there is a procedure for self-inspection and/or quality audit which regularly appraises the effectiveness and applicability of the Quality Assurance system."

This requirement clearly applies to transfusion organizations and it is, therefore, a statutory requirement that a documented audit program is developed and implemented.

Types of audit

There are several different types of GMP audit, each of which have a different function. These are as follows:

– *Self-inspection audits* are carried out in a section of an organization by staff within the area being audited. This is mainly to check that GMP policies are being carried out and to prevent complacency developing within the area.

– *Internal audits* are also carried out within the organization, but are carried out by trained staff who have no responsibility for the area being audited. This type of auditing is intended to provide systematic evidence of regulatory compliance and to provide the organization's management with information for future planning for GMP improvement and training.

– *External audit* is carried out by people from outside the organization, such as external audit companies, providing an objective assessment of the organization's quality system. A rather more stressful type of external audit is carried by inspectors from regulatory bodies. For example, in the UK, all transfusion centers were inspected by the UK Medicines Control Agency during 1992 or 1993.

– *Vendor audits* are carried out by an organization to inspect the suppliers of key components to ensure that quality specifications are met. For example, plasma fractionators must now carry out vendor audits of all suppliers of plasma to ensure that it is collected and tested in an approved manner.

Full details of the principles of GMP auditing are discussed elsewhere [5]. The rest of this brief review will concentrate on the role and benefits of internal audits within a transfusion organization.

Value of internal audits

A successful and well managed audit has a number of benefits, in addition to meeting statutory obligations. These benefits include the following:

– *Preparation for inspection by regulatory authorities* is of great benefit to staff so that they are exposed to GMP auditing before inspections by regulatory bodies. A program of GMP audits of regional transfusion centers in Scotland and Northern Ireland certainly helped to prepare for visits by a medicines inspector from the UK Medicines Control Agency.

– *Provides objective evidence of GMP compliance* which can allow staff and managers to assess the quality of their work and to plan and carry out necessary remedial action.

– *Encourages quality improvement* by elimination of GMP deficiencies and by ensuring that good ideas implemented in one area can be praised and then spread throughout the organization. It is essential to note that an effective quality audit will highlight the good points as well as the bad points detected during the audit.

– *Promotes self-criticism and self-improvement* by detecting areas of activity which are poorly understood or have been overlooked by the staff concerned.

– *Should result in cost savings* if wasteful practices can be identified and eliminated.

Requirements for a successful internal audit

There are a number of requirements which must be followed if an internal audit program is to be carried out successfully and maximum benefit is to be gained from each audit. These essential requirements are summarized briefly as follows:

– *Careful planning prior to the audit* is absolutely essential to ensure that attention is given to important aspects of the operation. If this is not done, the auditors may lack understanding of the area being audited and this may lead to a superficial, unstructured audit with limited value to managers and one which is not accepted by the people working in the area audited. The planning process will include the following points:

- Consult relevant documentation (SOPs, specifications, policies, regulations) relating to the area being audited.
- Consult any previous audit reports.
- Consult any inspection report from a regulatory body.
- Generate an audit check list.
- Ensure that relevant staff will be present during the audit.

– *Careful execution of the audit*, is clearly of crucial significance. A poorly executed audit will not provide valuable information and may undermine the validity of any conclusions. A well executed audit will include the following points.

- The audit must be carried out by trained auditor(s).
- The audit must be carried out objectively.
- The audit must concentrate on major issues such as validation of methods, availability of SOPs, accuracy of Documentation, effectiveness of cleaning, training, etc.
- Ensure accuracy of audit conclusions by discussion with staff being audited.
- Some type of scoring system should be adopted to indicate the degree of severity of any deficiencies noted.
- The confidence of the staff being audited should be achieved by ensuring that their comments are listened to and, where relevant, included in the audit report.

– *A thorough follow-up* is essential following each audit, in order to ensure that the conclusions from the audit are documented and that effective remedial action is taken. This phase is the most important stage of any audit and will include the following:

- A verbal report of the major conclusions from the audit should be given at the time of the audit.
- A detailed written report should be generated by the auditor within a short period after the completion of the audit. This report will identify deficiencies in procedure, in documentation, in training and in resources and facilities. The report should also advise of good points found during the audit. The report should then be circulated to all relevant managers and to the staff who were audited.
- The manager responsible should then ensure that a program of remedial action is developed to deal with the critical points which are raised, with particular attention being paid to the most serious deficiencies noted by the auditors.
- The adequacy of the planned remedial action should be agreed with the auditor.
- A record should be kept of the remedial action taken. When this is completed, the full audit file should be collated and the audit declared closed.

Scheduling of audits

Audits need to be thorough and should not normally take more than 1-3 days to complete. Thus, the audit program for an organization will be divided into manageable sections and should aim to cover all significant parts of the organization over a 1-2 year period. This will involve a phased program which can be published well in advance. It is generally not a good idea to arrive unannounced to perform an audit, because this leads to a significant lack of trust between the auditor and the staff of the area being audited. For this reason, it is strongly advised that the audit program is circulated well in advance of the planned audit dates.

Conclusion

It is clear that blood transfusion centers must adopt the same standards of GMP as apply to any other pharmaceutical manufacturer. Codes of Good Manufacturing Practice now apply to transfusion organizations and these must be implemented and enforced. Although each donation is considered to be a separate "batch" by regulatory authorities, it is essential that blood and blood products are manufactured and tested using standardized, reproducible methods which are fully developed, documented and controlled via an effective quality system. It is an essential requirement of any quality system that effective programs are developed for validation and audit of all key systems.

An integrated and structured validation program will cover and document the key components of the entire transfusion operation, notably:

- Pre-commissioning validation of new manufacturing methods, new assay methods, new equipment and new premises.

- Regular routine validation of key equipment.
- Routine monitoring and validation of the performance of manufacturing methods and laboratory assays.
- Microbiological monitoring is also a key component of the validation program.

All areas of transfusion practice must be subjected to regular audit by trained auditors who will check for compliance with accepted features of GMP including documentation, standardization, record keeping, cleaning, training and validation.

Audits must be systematic, objective, well planned and well documented. A detailed record must be made of the outcome of each audit and a written record must be made of remedial action taken.

Acknowledgements

Grateful thanks are offered to Miss Linda Burns for her patient typing of the manuscript and to Mr. Tony Jones for producing the high quality of slides used during the presentation. Thanks are also duo to Mrs. Ida Dickson, Dr. Katherine Reid, Mr. Bob Howieson, Mr. Martin Bruce and Mr. John Scott for helpful discussions which helped to formulate some of the ideas used in this manuscript.

References

1. Ad Hoc Working Party on Biotechnology/Pharmacy. Note for Guidance: Medicinal products derived from human blood and plasma. Commission of the European Communities Ref. 111/8379/89-EN, 1992.
2. Commission of the European Communities. Rules governing medicinal products in the European Community. Vol. IV. Good Manufacturing Practice for medicinal products. Office for Official Publications of European Communities, 1992.
3. Guidelines for the Blood Transfusion Service, 2nd Ed. HMSO Publications, 1993.
4. Council of Europe. Guide to the preparation use and quality assurance of blood components. Council of Europe Press, Strasbourg 1992.
5. Sharp J. Good Manufacturing Practice. Philosophy and applications. Interpharm Press, Buffalo Grove, IL, 1991.
6. Steinhorn L. GMP Quality audit manual for healthcare manufacturers and their suppliers. Interpharm Press, Buffalo Grove, IL, 1991.
7. Oakland J.S. Total Quality Management. Butterworth Heinemann, Oxford, 1990.

QUALITY CONTROL AND RELEASE PROCEDURES FOR PRODUCTS DERIVED FROM HUMAN BLOOD OR HUMAN PLASMA APPLICATION TO PASTEURIZED PLASMA

B. Flan, T. Burnouf, J.J. Huart

Quality control of products derived from blood or plasma, which are considered as medicines of human origin at the European level since the Directive 89/381-June 1989 [1] (extending the scope of Directive 65/65 [2] on medicines for human use) was published, is a key element in guaranteeing their efficacy and safety. It involves issues common to all drugs and specific points to consider with regard to the particularity of the source material and the processing steps involved during manufacture, i.e. virus inactivation. The aim of this paper is not to give an extensive overview of Quality Control (QC) procedures, as they are largely described in the existing regulation; examples include GMP rules [3] as extended recently to products derived from human blood and plasma [4,5]. Rather, our intention is to focus on some issues of QC procedures that are specifically related to the manufacturing of safe and efficacious blood products. The approach developed in the Centre Régional de Transfusion Sanguine (CRTS) of Lille for the manufacturing of virus-inactivated pasteurized plasma (VIP) will illustrate our topic. The manufacturing process of VIP and its validation in terms of process and virus safety have been described by Burnouf-Radosevich et al. [6-8].

The role of QC can be summarized as a way to guarantee that all the *incomings and outgoings* in the manufacture of a medicinal product are of a recognized quality, compatible with a product that will achieve both clinical efficacy and safety. This requirement to ensure the QC aspects of the manufacturing process leads to the basic notions of 1) traceability; 2) documentation; and 3) release.

Traceability

The requirement for traceability is an important feature, common to the whole pharmaceutical field (and in general to all industrial processes engaged in a quality approach). The traceability of incoming materials is relatively easy to set up in terms of batches of raw materials, chromatography supports, filters and so on. In the case of blood or plasma derived products (BP) the traceability to the source material (plasma donations) requires the setting of a complex record keeping system to correctly handle the documentation allowing the complete traceability from donors to batches of BP and from batches to donors. In this connection, for the manufacture of VIP, the CRTS of Lille has implemented a computerized system: Before commencing production of a given batch, the numbers of each blood donation collected at the Lille Blood Bank, are recorded one by one under a pre-established batch number by means of bar code reading (note: In France the number of donations is restricted to 100 per batch for this specific pooled product). The blood bags for this batch are stored in a closed, temperature-controlled container, identified by the batch number; this batch number is also bar-coded. When starting the batch production, the operator checks the batch number, records it by bar-code reading and the blood bags are recorded one by one before the thawing step. The central computer which controls the overall manufacturing process, automatically records the batch number and all the steps of the manufacturing process, storing the most important data (washings, addition of stabilizers, virus inactivation, ultrafiltration) through a magnetic system for identification of the containers and equipments used during the process. This system allows easy traceability of donors to batch, from QC data of the blood donations (such as the blood screening tests) to the final release of the batch. The extension of this system to all the products manufactured at the CRTS of Lille is in progress; however, it is mostly dependant upon harmonization of identification systems (bar-code) for blood bags at the national (or international) level. Recent developments in coding systems may facilitate progress in this specific area. This issue is quite fundamental to the safe handling of traceability from donors to batches of plasma derived products and could possibly be extended to the patients receiving the product.

Documentation

QC procedures must cover all the steps of the manufacturing process, from raw materials to the final release of the end product (and also to the handling of complaints). The recognized quality of all the incomings must first be documented and, secondly, accepted by a properly qualified person. The documentation covers many issues that can be summarized in quality standards leading to acceptance criteria. These quality standards are either general, directly issued from the regulatory background or specific to the product: Defined during the development of the product and described in the registration file. Table 1 illustrates the definition of these standards of quality. The development of a new product is a key phase for the setting of QC procedures. It include at least:

- The definition of the quality of raw materials (chemicals, chromatography supports, ...) and acceptable limits that have to be met for good manufacturing.
- The definition of the specifications to allow the final release of the batches, ensuring safety and efficacy, as related to the performance of the production process itself.
- The process validation which leads to the selection of production parameters which needs to be monitored routinely, thus ensuring consistency in production. It will also determine, if applicable, the frequency of any periodic revalidation.

Table 1. Definition of quality standards and acceptance criteria for quality control.

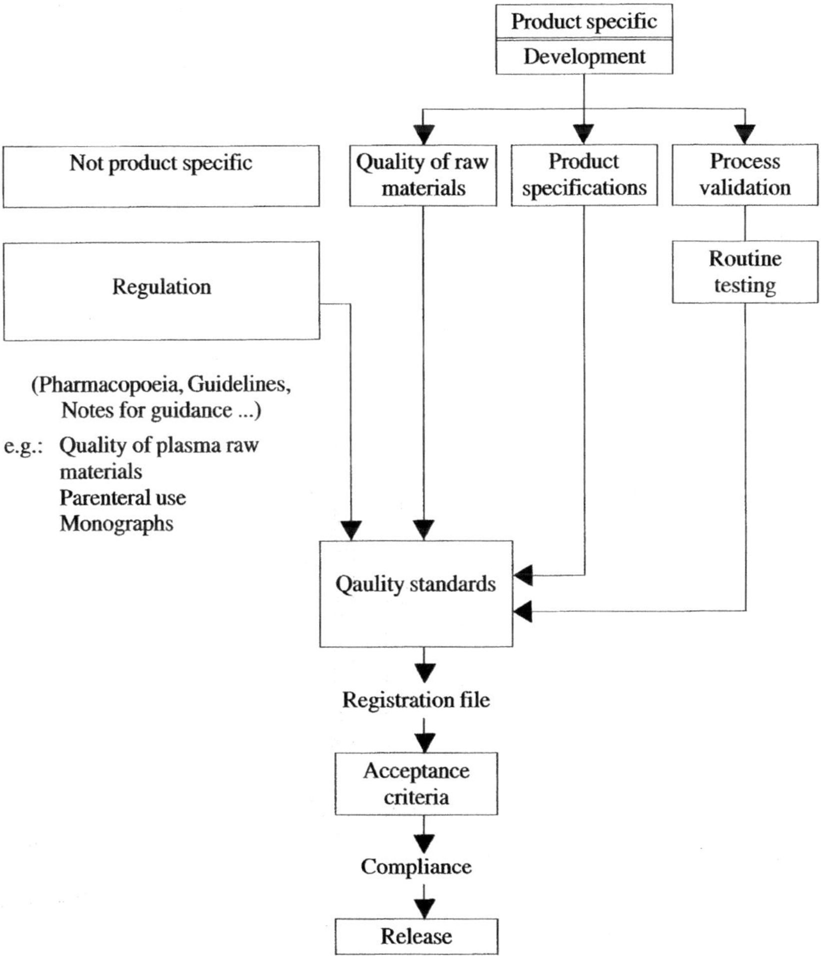

Release

The release of any incoming or outcoming material has to be handled by a properly qualified person whose role is to guarantee 1) that the available information to determine the quality properties of the material allows correct evaluation of its quality; and 2) that the material complies with the pre-established quality standards.

Table 2. General scheme of quality control of blood derivatives.

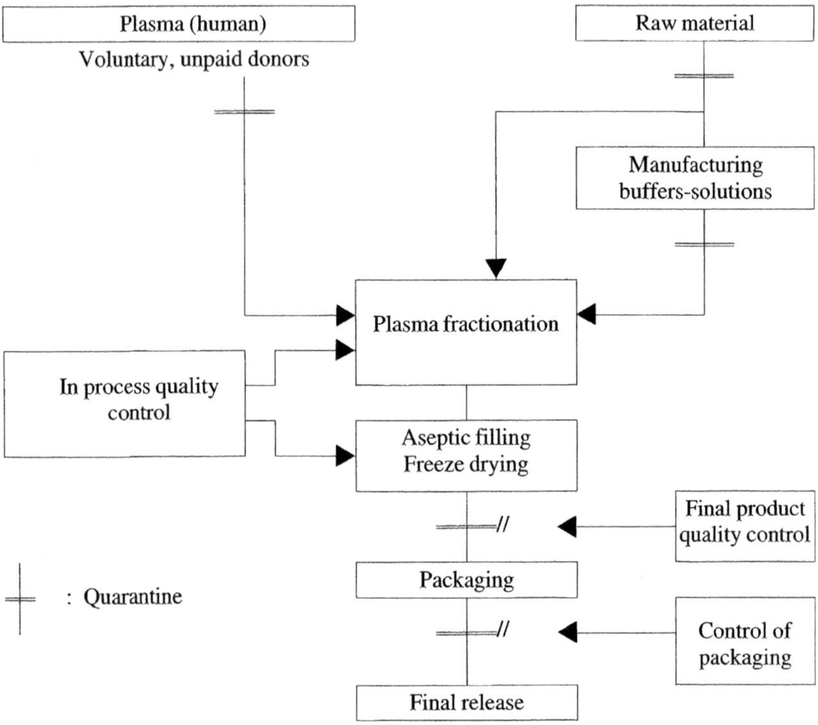

Table 3. Definition of quarantine and sequence of events associated with quarantine.

⇓

Quarantine

- Procedures for entry
- Sampling:
  - Sampling plans
  - Method
- Analysis
- Documentation
- Expertise of documentation
- Release
- Procedures for outgoing

⇓

Quality control/Quality assurance relationships

The Quality Assurance (QA) program represents a strong prerequisite for an efficient QC program. The conditions in which the product is manufactured, are indeed one of the key parameters for good quality: Compliance with GMP rules must first be guaranteed.

The involvement of QC in the acceptance of any incoming or outgoing material is summarized on Table 2 and leads to the fundamental notion of quarantine (physical or not) which is the state of a product which quality is being explored before release. A general scheme for quarantine is described on Table 3, every step mentioned in this table must be carefully handled by adequate procedures.

Except for the special case of raw materials which must be identified in each and every container, QC relies on testing performed on samples that have to be taken in a statistical way. The homogeneity of the batches to be controlled is the basis of an efficient QC, completed by suitable sampling plans. The sampling can also focus on sensitive points of critical steps, for example, in the case of sterility testing for the validation of the aseptic filling step. These notions illustrate the total interdependence and complementary of QC and QA.

The key issues for QC at the different steps of the process are summarized in Tables 4-7. Additional to physicochemical and biological activity testings, the bacteriological contamination must be monitored during the process through QC of raw material; sterilization of buffers or solutions, careful monitoring of in-

Table 4. Raw materials quality control.

- Chemicals
- Filter aids
- Chromatography supports

Key issues for quality control:

- Physicochemical identification
- Physicochemical characterization (sample)
  - Purity
  - Impurities
- Bacteriological quality (sample)
  - Bacterial counts
  - Endotoxin content (+/- pyrogen test)

Table 5. Quality control of buffers/solutions.

– Physicochemical testing	⟹	Compliance with manufacturing formula
– Testing for sterility		
– Testing for pyrogens		
– Endotoxin content		

Table 6. In process quality control.

Monitoring of the manufacturing process

Physicochemical and biological activity testing (Cohn fractionation, chromatography, buffers, adjustment, viral inactivation ...)

Monitoring of the hygienic conditions for manufacture

- In process bacterial counts:
  - Starting material
  - Pre-sterile filtration
  - Key steps (storage, elution ...)
- Validation of the sanitization program: Limulus test (equipment, UF, chromatography ...) (+ absence of sanitizing agents after sanitization)
- In process testing for endotoxin content/pyrogens

Monitoring of aseptic conditions for filling

- Quality of air
- Monitoring of operators

Table 7. Final product quality control.

Safety

- Testing for sterility
- Animal testing:
  - Pyrogen test
  - Abnormal toxicity
  - Animal models
- Endotoxin content
- In vitro testing for
  - Prekallikrein activators
  - Thrombogenicity
  - Markers for activation
  - Viral markers
  - Haemagglutinins
  - Aluminium (albumin)

Efficacy: Active ingredient

- Quantitative:
  - Physicochemical testing (protein content)
  - Biological activity (coagulation factors, specific IgG)
- Qualitative:
  - Purity:
    - Electrophoresis
    - Molecular size distribution
    - Specific activity
  - Functional integrity (ratios: immunochemical (Ag)/biological activity)
  - Contaminants (proteins)

Formulation: Excipient(s)

- Suitability for intravenous administration: Osmolality, pH ...
- Dosage of excipient(s): Buffer, salts, stabilizers
- Dosage of adjuvant(s): Residual solvent, detergent, ethanol
- Water content in freeze-dried products

Table 8. Flow sheet of transfer of information for labelling and packaging.

QC Department

Batch documentation
- Process
- QC analysis

⇓

Authorization for packaging

⇓

Validation by head of QC

⇓

Information for labelling
- Batch No.
- Expiry date
- Potency
- No. of vials

⇓

Validation by head of QC

⇓

Packaging department

Automatic transfer to printers

⇓

Labelling and packaging

process bacteriological counts are major points to consider, reinforced by the fact that BP cannot be sterilized in their final container. Pyrogen tests in rabbits and endotoxin contamination must be performed and handled properly. The parameters listed in these tables can be directly monitored by analyses performed in QC laboratories, following procedures complying with Good Laboratory Practice (GLP). In the case of BP, submitted to virus inactivation treatments, the efficacy of the virus inactivation step(s), performed in process, as well as in the final container cannot be revealed by specific QC tests and must, hence, rely only on the strict relation to establish production parameters (or criteria) leading to a parametric release of this crucial step. The role of QC in this particular case is to confirm that the virus inactivation step has been performed according to the conditions that have been validated. In this respect, the virus inactivation of plasma at CRTS Lille, in the manufacturing of VIP is achieved by in-process heat treatment at 60°C for 10 hours in the liquid state. This step is performed in closed jacketed containers, in an isolated virus safe area, involving manual and automatic process controls which ensure safety; the computer system checks that the sequence of events has been completed before starting: Cleaning in place of the inactivation container, integrity, closure system, time, temperature. The double enveloped container, itself, is validated for its suitability to guarantee homogeneous heat treatment of the product. Post inactivation steps occur in the virus safe area. The conditions of the treatment have to be checked on every batch of BP; automatic systems provide an aid in the guarantee of reproducibility of a validated process.

Similarly, the guarantee for bacterial sterility of one batch is not achieved uniquely by the final product sterility testing. It is, like the virus inactivation step and, as mentioned in the pharmacopoeia, the result of compliance with GMP during the filling (and freeze drying) step.

The QC must also check the conformity of the packaging, the details for packaging being directly issued from QC. They include data like expiry date and potency of coagulation factors. In this connection, we have, in CRTS Lille, implemented the direct transmission of the details for labelling (expiry date, potency, specific activity, number of vials) from the QC department to the printing machines of the packaging department, without any retranscription of data according to the scheme (Table 8).

Every single step governs the continuation of the process, guaranteeing that only accepted batches are packaged with the correct information, validated by the head of the QC. The number of labels to be printed is also managed by this system, which represents another security step. The validation of the parameters for packaging by the head of the QC is required for the preparation of the packaging materials (leaflets, boxes, labels, ...) by the operators.

The final release of the batch takes place after ensuring the compliance of the overall documentation of the batch. Samples of end product, raw materials, plasma pools and some in-process samples must be retained for further analyses, for example, in case of complaints.

References

1. Council Directive 89/381/EEC of 14 June 1989, extending the scope of Directives 65/65/EEC and 75/319/EEC on the approximation of provisions laid down by law, regulation or administrative action relating to proprietary medicinal products and laying down special provisions for medicinal products derived from human blood or human plasma. O.J. No. L 181 of 28.6.89.
2. Council Directive 65/65/EEC of 26 January 1965 on the approximation of provisions laid down by law, regulation or administrative action relating to proprietary medicinal products. O.J. No. 22 of 9.2.65.
3. Commission of the European Communities. The rules governing medicinal products in the European Community. Good Manufacturing Practice for medicinal products, Vol. IV.
4. Medicinal products derived from human blood and plasma. Ad Hoc working party on Biotechnology/Pharmacy. Note for guidance III/8379/89-EN.
5. Manufacture of products derived from human blood or human plasma. Working party on control of medicines and inspections. Annex to the EC guide to GMP, III/3232/92-EN.
6. Burnouf-Radosevich M, Burnouf T, Huart JJ. A pasteurized therapeutic plasma. Infusionstherapie 1992;19:91-4.

7. Burnouf-Radosevich M, Burnouf T, Huart JJ. Development and experience of a pasteurization process for pooled fresh frozen plasma. In: Rivat C, Stolz JF (eds). Biotechnology of blood proteins. Proceedings of the 2nd INSERM international symposium, Nancy (France) 1992:16-8.
8. Burnouf-Radosevich M, Burnouf T, Huart JJ. Pasteurisation industrielle du plasma et critères de qualité. Rev Fr Transfus Hémobiol 1993;36:93-102.

A PLANT FOR THE MANUFACTURING OF VIRUS INACTIVATED PLASMA ACCORDING TO GMP-GUIDELINES

B. Kerner, P. Selosse

Introduction

Fresh Frozen Plasma (FFP) is prepared in blood banks throughout the world, as a separation product of whole blood. The viral safety of FFP depends on donor selection and screening. Despite implementation of measures a definite residual risk of virus transmission still remains. Estimates of residual risk vary, and depend upon the prevalence of infection within the country, the stability of the donor population and the sensitivity and specificity of the test kits used.

FFP can now be substituted by a solvent-detergent treated plasma [1-4] which has demonstrated both its efficacy and safety in a number of clinical trials [5-8].

The solvent-detergent inactivation step occurs as a part of the production process and not as a final treatment of the finished product. This non-terminal step raises concerns about possible recontamination by the manufacturing environment after virus inactivation.

These concerns and the avoidance of this possibility were the basis for design specification of the manufacturing facility for Octaplas.

Octaplas is a virus-inactivated plasma for transfusion produced by the solvent-detergent treatment of FFP. Octaplas is produced using 350 l pools of plasma of specific origin, often as part of a self-sufficiency program.

Good Manufacturing Practice (GMP) is a vital part of self-sufficiency, if guarantees of non-contamination of plasma and return of country-specific plasma is to be achieved. Segregation of plasma is facilitated by a system of colour coding and by total production of only one batch at a time. This segregation of virus inactivated product from non virus inactivated product by means of environmental measures is the subject of this paper.

Preparation of Octaplas (Table 1)

FFP units of identical blood group are thawed rapidly in a tank. The plasma pool is then filtered to remove small-sized particles and aggregated materials. The solvent-detergent mixture [1% tri(n-butyl)phosphate (TNBP) and 1% triton X-100] is added and homogenized by stirring.

Table 1.

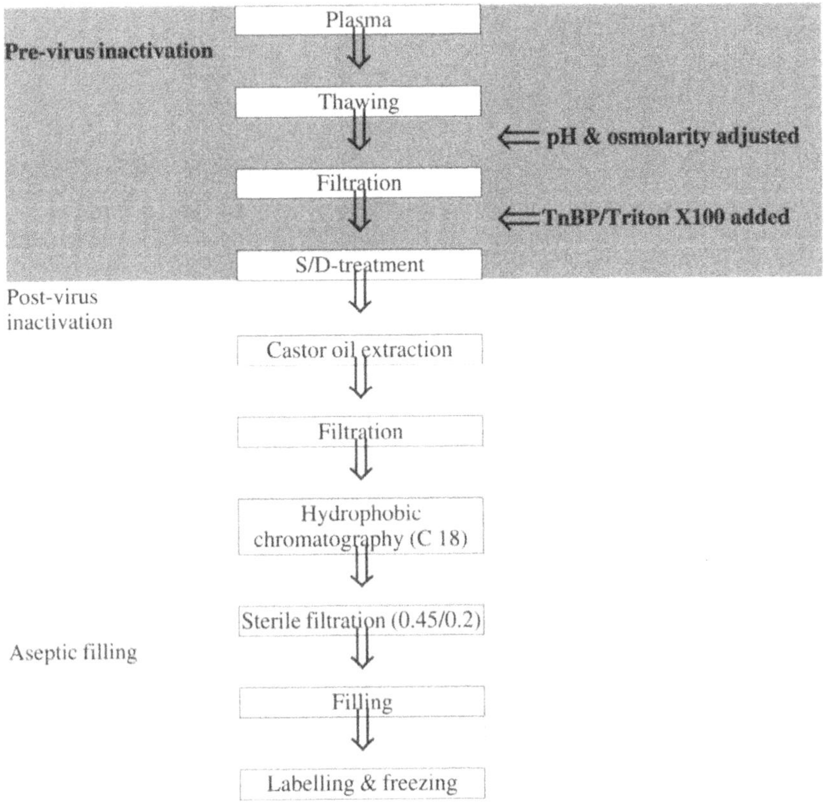

After a specified time this is transferred into the virus inactivation tank in a specially equipped virus-free area, and virus inactivation takes place.

After completion of this step the product is regarded as virus inactivated and all further manipulations are performed under virus safe conditions. The subsequent steps include the removal of the virus inactivation reagents by extraction with castor oil, a further filtration and preparative reversed phase chromatography.

In the final stage the product is sterile-filtered and filled under aseptic conditions into sterile PVC bags. After the bags have been sealed they are labelled, vacuum-packed and snapfrozen.

GMP considerations (Figure 1)

Safety against recontamination can be achieved by a production environment that allows only a unidirectional materials flow (Figure 2). All products, materials and personnel have to be lifted over physical barriers.

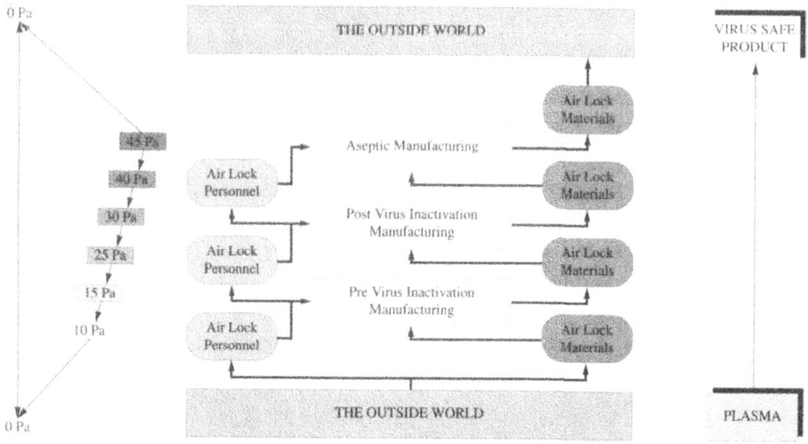

Figure 1. Good manufacturing practice.

There is a physical separation of the pre-virus inactivation areas and the area for post-virus inactivation operations . Separation is achieved by solid walls. As an additional feature an area for the aseptic filling is provided, because the product cannot be sterilized in the final container. Plasma moves from the pre-virus inactivation area to the post-virus inactivation area and aseptic filling area in one direction only.

Personnel can enter each area only via air locks. Access to these areas is strictly limited through the use of an ID-card system. In the air locks clothing is changed and personnel undergo hygiene procedures. All materials are entered or removed via air locks. There is no access to the different production areas except via a multistage air lock system.

To prevent the entry of any contaminants, the whole area is maintained under positive air pressure. Inside the production area there is an air pressure gradient from 45 Pascal against atmospheric pressure in aseptic manufacturing to 30 Pascal in the post-virus inactivation area to 15 Pascal in the pre-virus inactivation area. This air pressure gradient is maintained and recorded during production. These data are an important part of environmental control in the production documents.

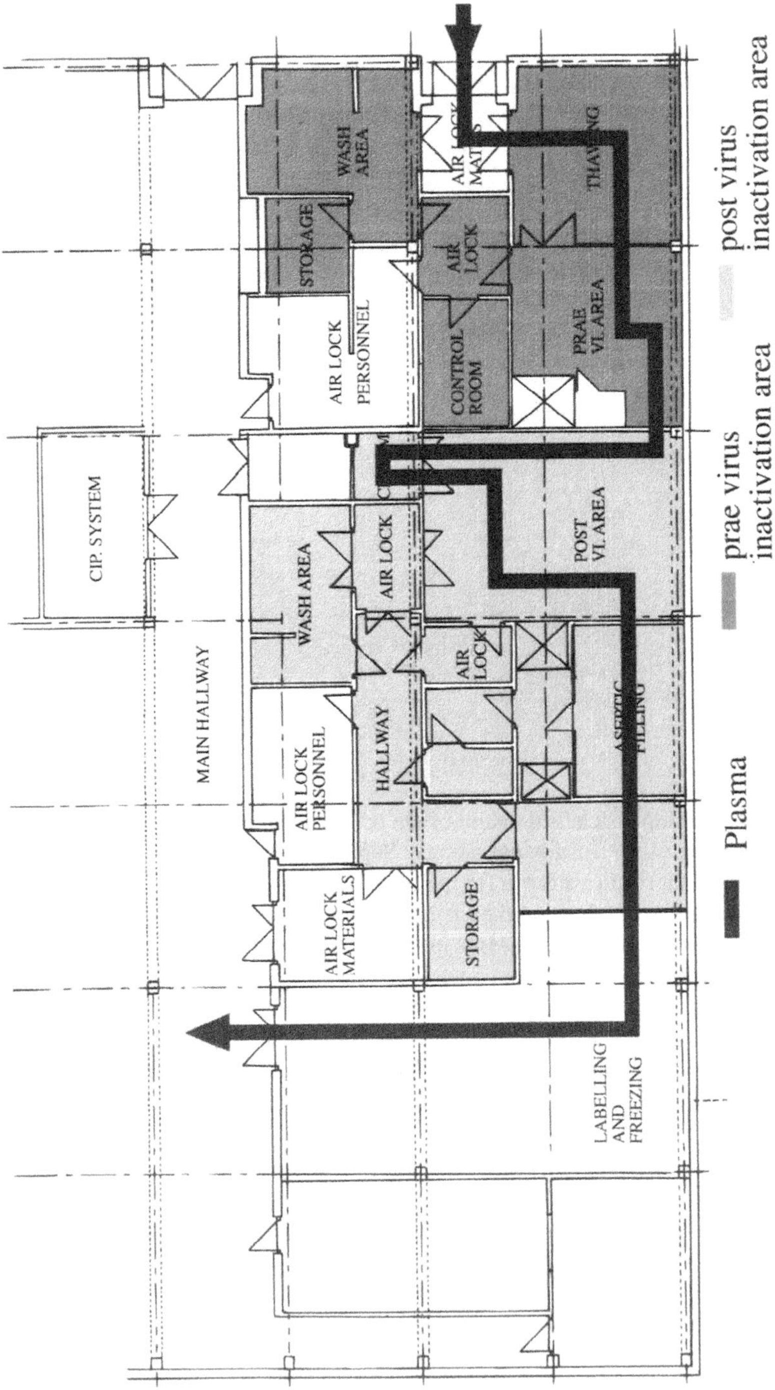
WASH AREA
STORAGE
AIR LOCK PERSONNEL
AIR LOCK
CONTROL ROOM
PRAE VI. AREA
CIP. SYSTEM
MAIN HALLWAY
WASH AREA
AIR LOCK
POST VI. AREA
HALLWAY
AIR LOCK PERSONNEL
AIR LOCK MATERIALS
STORAGE
LABELLING AND FREEZING
Plasma
prae virus inactivation area
post virus inactivation area

In addition, air is filtered by HEPA-filters and conditioned with regard to temperature and humidity. Cleanliness classes are:

- Class A for the aseptic manufacturing
- Class B in the surrounding area
- Class C in the processing areas

The post-virus inactivation area has a separate air-handling system which prevents air mixture with that of the pre-virus inactivation area.

Summary

The above environmental standards, namely layout of the facility, air handling and materials flow, are only part of GMP.

They only are meaningful when the rest of the system such as raw material and finished product specifications, in-process testing, personnel, organization, equipment and quality control, also follow proper GMP.

In the case of Octaplas manufacture in the Vienna facility, a system of Quality Assurance supports GMP.

All applied procedures have been validated and the premises have been subject to inspection and qualification.

The results of one year's operation with hundreds of batches demonstrate that the concept is effective as no recontamination has been observed.

References

1. Piquet Y, Janvier G, Selosse P, et al. In: Smit Sibinga CTh, Das PC, Cash JD (eds). Transfusion Medicine: Fact and Fiction. Kluwer Academic Publ., Dordrecht/Boston/London, 1991:189-90.
2. Horowitz B, Bonomo R, Prince AM, Chin SN, Brotman B, Shulman RW. Solvent/Detergent-treated plasma: A virus-inactivated substitute for fresh frozen plasma. Blood 1992;79:826-31.
3. Hellstern P, Sachse H, Schwinn H, Oberfrank K. Manufacture and in vitro characterization of a solvent/detergent-treated human plasma. Vox Sang 1992;63:178-85.
4. Piquet Y, Janvier G, Selosse P, et al. Virus inactivation of fresh frozen plasma by a solvent detergent procedure: Biological results. Vox Sang 1992;63:251-6.
5. Hellstern P, Larbig E, Walz GA, Thüringen W, Oberfrank K. Prospective study on efficacy and tolerability of solvent/detergent-treated plasma in intensive care unit patients. Infusionstherapie und Transfusionsmedizin, S. Karger 1993;20(Suppl 2):16-8.
6. Inbal A, Epstein O, Blickstein D, Kornbrot N, Brenner B, Martinowitz U. Evaluation of solvent/detergent treated plasma in the management of patients with hereditary and acquired coagulation disorders. Blood Coagulation and Fibrinolysis 1993;4:599-604.
7. Tocci LJ, Napychank PA, Cable RG, Snyder EL. The effect of solvent/detergent-treated plasma on stored platelet concentrates. Transfusion 1993;33:145-9.
8. Solheim BG, Mohre B, Noddeland H, et al. The use of Octaplas in patients undergoing open heart surgery. Submitted.

BAR CODING IN HEALTH CARE: THE NEEDS OF THE BLOOD BANKS

H. Oehlmann

Good Manufacturing Practice (GMP) rules, similar to the TQM program for industry, have been worked out and gradually introduced in order to achieve a high quality standard in health care. Reliability plays an important role in this and is directly linked to the traceability of products, samples and events. Bar code has now been used successfully for over a decade in an attempt to achieve reliable identification. The reliability rate of bar code is several million to one, compared with error rates of 300 to one for manual identification.

In blood transfusion technology, the link between the donor blood bag and samples has been traditionally achieved using Codabar for so-called set labels (Figure 1). These contain a set of vignettes, from which partial labels with the same number are attached to the relevant samples, so that a connection between these can be maintained.

Internationally, other symbologies such as Code 39 are used. For internal purposes this is irrelevant, but a uniform data structure and symbology should be maintained.

Figure 1. The set label.

Figure 2. The product label with data in Codabar structure and in ISBT 128 Codabar structure.

Nowadays, more and more interconnections arise as a result of the exchange of products in blood transfusion. Initial products are transported from one point to another for further processing. Blood products, the origin of which must be demonstrable, are transported to hospitals.

- *Traceability* is the decisive factor for reliability throughout the whole logistical chain from the donor to sample taking, analysis, etc. to interim storage and use. Internal standards are no longer sufficient to guarantee this. The International Society of Blood Transfusion (ISBT) has announced an extension of the current regulations in a standard in order to cover the requirements for additional information in the data structure and to remove the restrictions of Codabar.
- *The ISBT 128 standard* has been designed in such a way that in the transitional period the traditional Codabar structure can be used, as well as the ISBT 128 code, which consists of data and Code 128. A significant criterion of ISBT 128 is the concatenation of data fields, which is possible with the so-called data identifier as a prefix to each data field.
  Handling and reliability of the linear Code 28 is improved even more by the use of the 2-dimensional Codablock F128. All data is read and transmitted simultaneously and errors in the reading of code fields on different products is thus excluded. The working groups of different countries submit the standard to their national committees so that it can become legally binding.

CEN, ANSI and ISO

The "Comité Européen de Normalisation" (CEN) in Europe, the "American Normalisation Institute" (ANSI) and FACT, the "Federation of Automated Coding Technologies" cooperate to achieve international reliability and thus traceability, which is in everyone's interest for the improvement of health care.

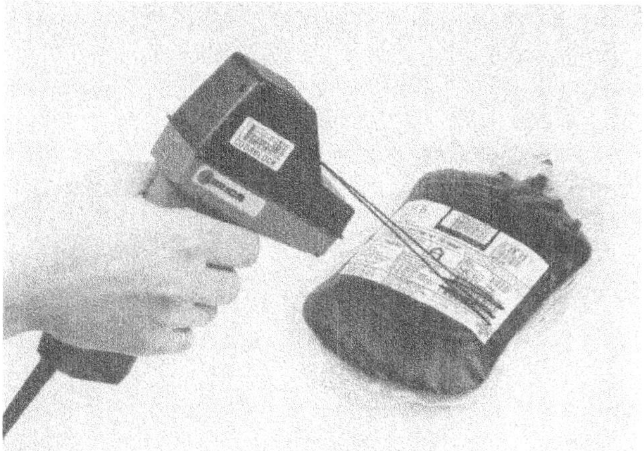

Figure 3. The reading of Codabar linear and ISBT 128 in two-dimensional Codablock.

How is the transition to the ISBT 128 standard possible?

Transition is achieved through the data structure, which allows parallelism between traditional and extended data structure. In addition, Codabar can be used together with ISBT 128 in Codablock F128 to save space on a label. The data can be read in traditional form as well as completely from the data carrier label, depending on which equipment or data base is available (Figure 2). Codablock acts here as a symbology converter so that available equipment can still be used for printing and reading.

- *The bar code reader as a converter* can always be used whenever a data base has not yet been established to store data for traceability purposes. Here, decoders can be used, which are able to translate information coded in Codabar, Code 128 or Codablock 128 to the structure of the respective data base, but maintaining the same data content (Figure 3).

Identcode with standard data structure is indispensable for reliability in transfusion medicine technology

Long-term experience has shown that the label plays a decisive role as a data carrier. In such case, the data structure is more significant than the symbology, which in future must have alphanumeric characters in order to meet the requirements of health care and transfusion medicine for quality in data and information flow.

DISCUSSION

P.A. Hoppe and P.C. Das

P.A. Hoppe (Bethesda, VA, USA): Mr. Caglioti, in relation to training and resources for training do you have any estimate of what percentage of a blood centre budget might properly be allocated to training?

T. Caglioti (Raritan, NJ, USA): The figure that should be targeted is about 2 to 3 per cent of your total payroll budget to be spent on training[1]. That is for a successful Total Quality Management organisation.

P.A. Hoppe: Do you have any idea how that figure compares to the amount most blood centers spend currently?

T. Caglioti: Sofar, from what we have seen in the US most blood centers are not quite there, yet. They are somewhere below 1 per cent if not below 0.5 per cent.

B.M. Eggen (Trondheim, N): I have two remarks, that I would like you to comment on. First, I have looked upon blood banking as a medical discipline up to now, but my impression from today is that it is turning into a pharmaceutical industry. Secondly with regard to Norway, we have a scarce population, we have long distances and we have about 60 hospitals with blood banks doing both collection and processing. Is this a situation that we have to change dramatically?

B.T. Teague (Houston, TX, USA): Since I am obviously committed to a service program rather than a product, I feel obligated to respond to that. I do believe we can have the best of both worlds, if we are very careful about how we do it. I do believe that there are processes, which can improve the quality of service, that we now provide and I believe those are very worthwhile to achieve. They must, however, be achieved without losing the human aspect of this profession. So, I believe very strongly in the need to have processes to document what we are doing and continuously strive to do better. I am not sure a totally harmless trans-

1. Training (ed) 1993. Industry Report, November 1993;30:43-5.

fusion will ever be possible under the current restraints, but we must try to achieve to get there. We must do the best we can. We will never get there, if we do not continue to improve the processes by which we do various things. But again we cannot lose the human response because there are some things from a human touch that simply are amenable or are not possible through a mechanical processing such as pharmaceuticals. So, I think we have to blend both, we cannot ignore either one.

P.A. Hoppe: I would like to add a balancing opinion to that. I agree in part, but I think considering blood "a product" is a little bit like the weather. It is inevitable; there is not a lot you can do about it. The "service" argument has been lost; blood is clearly considered a product. I think we are going to be better off if we put our effort into addressing those issues that relate to GMP for products. In regard to the issue of whether or not increased Quality Assurance requirements are going to drive some small operations out of business, I am afraid I have to agree that in the interest of efficiency and economy we surely will have to reconsider whether there needs to be regionalization of services in many areas. I would suspect that in a country the size of Norway, 60 centers may be more than is optimal if you want to achieve the highest quality operation at a reasonable cost. It is an issue that is very big both in the USA and other places, because people feel strongly about continuing the services they have provided. However, it appears that better quality products are more easily achieved in larger volume facilities most of the time.

B.A. Kerner (Vienna, A): I might just reiterate the same point as we start looking at outcomes in healthcare in general. There is a point where you need to do a certain critical volume in order to be able to do procedures reliably, where systems and processes are no different. When you have your cardiac bypass you like to go to a place that is doing 40 or 50 or more rather than some hospital that is doing 10 a year. The outcomes are better, the mortalities are lower etc. I think the same is true in blood bank processing. You need to be doing it every day on a regular basis to understand how the system works to be able to manage it in an appropriate way. Regionalization is certainly a trend happening worldwide. So, I am sure it will continue.

P.C. Das (Groningen, NL): Dr. Cuthbertson, you mentioned that the United States is very lucky to have the FDA as a centralized organization, whereas we heard our American colleagues were not happy with the FDA although for different reasons. The European situation, however, is very fragmented, for example in England you need the permission of the National Institute of Biological Standards. In the Netherlands you need permission from the Ministry of Health and in Germany from other institutes. Is this correct, it is so fragmented in Europe?

B. Cuthbertson (Edinburgh, UK): In terms of health care release there is no system in the UK at all. There are pros and cons of the FDA system in that the FDA licenses kits. That gives users some kind of protection legally against any mismanufacturing by the manufacturers. The con of that clearly is that it can mean that the release of kits is held up. For example recombinant kits; kits including recombinant HIV were used in the European scene before they were used in America, and they had demonstrable sensitivity improvement. So, there are pros and cons for a regulated system. There are already movements within the EEC to think about a similar system and the UK are considering whether there might be fit bodies to take on this kind of role.

E. Vasconcelos (Lisbon, P): Mr. Teague, I am wondering if the blood banking work is regarded as a service, if it is still under the consumer protection or product liability act.

B.T. Teague: In the United States nearly every state has a state law that says the provision of blood constitutes a service, not a sale. Therefore, there is not an implicit strict liability. That is the legal definition by state and is fairly uniform across the states and is called "a blood shield statute". I think the argument of whether it is a service or whether it is a product, as my very respected colleague Ann Hoppe, says this is probably moot. The other reason I contend we should obtain the service aspect is to not lose the personal touch. Clearly in the States the law is the FDA and the law calls it a product. That is the reason you saw product in my presentation repeatedly. I just do not want any of us to lose the personal aspect. The plaintive lawyers in the States will quickly argue that since you call it a product, you should be held strictly liable, regardless of what happens you should be held liable. Under the current law blood banks are not held liable unless they are found to be negligent, which is a huge difference. Legislation in the United States is a major driving force in blood banking and I am not sure that is true in many other countries.

C.Th. Smit Sibinga (Groningen, NL): I just would like to reenforce these statements. Of course, we have heard much about pharmaceutical terminology, pharmaceutical technology, pharmaceutical approaches. They indeed do have an important role to play today and in the future within the field of transfusion medicine bridging the donor community to the patient. The point which has arisen is, that the medical field has been a bit overenthusiastic immediately adapting to this terminology and forgetting about the background, which is indeed the service. We are dealing with a product produced by the donor. Prof. Gormley has quite clearly stated, that the donor is not a factory producing a source material. He is a volunteer, preferably on a non-renumerated basis, who is sharing some tissue, a living transplant, which we within the blood bank community have the task and the obligation to further process according to pharmaceutical principles. That is where GMP comes in. That is where we have to change our thinking and where we can learn much from our pharmaceutical colleagues. They have a definite role to play within the blood bank community. However, that does not change the origin of the material, the human blood as a gift; it does not change the end product still being a living tissue or a functional protein. Despite all the formulations, specifically in fractionation, into freeze-dried virus-inactivated powders which can be redissolved and injected intravenously etc., it does not change the origin. It does not change human blood or its constituents into a medicinal product, a pharmacon, but the approaches to it are definitely pharmaceutical. I am quite convinced that they will increase over the years. We have a lot to learn in our behaviour. One of the major words which is the red thread through the symposium is teaching, teaching, teaching. We have to educate ourselves, which is the whole purpose of this symposium.

Dr. Oehlmann, fascinating of course to try to change a system for the future coming from Codabar, which was instituted in 1977 by the Committee on Commonality in Blood Banking Administration into System 128. However, the problem is: How do you see the conversion into 128 without falling into clerical errors in a day-to-day routine, where there is Codabar instituted with stocks of labels, with products being labelled, to be stored long term and short term.

H. Oehlmann (Neu-Anspach, D): This is a fair question and indeed that is the reason that in ISBT the working party made a proposal to look for migration parts between the old symbol and the new symbol. Not only the symbol used, but also the new codification method, which includes the data identifier structure which increases the all over security incredibly. If you would just change from Codabar label to Code 128 the analyzing machine would not read it; that is a fact. But those who intend to go with the future trend could without any additional costs use the new technology and so open the migration parts.

C.Th. Smit Sibinga: It is not only the codes and the labels, but the reading is even more essential. Therefore, the programming, the software in our computers then needs a major change to convert the one system to the other.

B. Oehlmann: Yes, this is a matter of the database and it is just a matter of checking the identifiers.

C.Th. Smit Sibinga: Is it that simple? A barcode system interrelates to basically every part of a program in automation from the very onset of the donor registration to the very end in the clinic. All these have to be converted.

B. Oehlmann: Yes, you are completely right, but you can do a lot in preprocessing, module per module. The basic question is what does industry or what do the blood banks have in mind for the future.

P.A. Hoppe: I would just comment from the USA standpoint. We are enthusiastic about the Code 128. It would be very disappointing if the rest of the world does not also adopt it, because it will mean a change for all of our blood banks.

We are willing to go through that change, because we think the long term benefits of having a uniform system with sufficient capacity for the future is extremely important. There have been a lot of discussions primarily among the data specialists; perhaps not enough of the blood bank people have been involved. I would urge blood center staff to get in touch with the data processing staff attending the ISBT meetings to learn what the answers are, because the potential problems have been thought through rather carefully. Everyone admits there are some hurdles that we are going to have to get past, but people believe we can achieve uniformity. There is such a large reward to be reaped, that we ought to all cooperate in getting the job done.

B. Oehlmann: I think there are features involved, which are not yet existing: There are no worldwide unique identifications of blood centers. So, that decision has to be taken and agreed upon.

K. Sazama (Sacramento, CA, USA): I have had the privilege of participating in discussions about Code 128 as a member of the American Association of Blood Banks committee, the Information Systems Committee. There will be an open discussion about these very questions at the annual meeting this year (1993) in October. I will share with you that I concur with dr. Smit Sibinga's comments and have raised these questions myself about the impact on some of the smaller self-sustaining information systems in some blood centers and transfusion services in the US. This is not an inconsiderable change that is being proposed. Although there are participants on the AABB committee from a number of major US-based computer companies, looking at the issues and trying to help to solve some of the difficulties with the proposed symbology change, one should be cognizant of the fact that it represents a major change. There are many features of Code 128 that make it a desirable change. Probably that observation is biased because, when we try to transfuse blood in non-English speaking countries, it is clearly beneficial to have common bar code symbology. There has been an enormous voluntary effort on the part of many blood bankers in the United States to try to reach these kind of questions and provide them the obvious support of the US FDA as well. But I think these are the kinds of questions that need to be raised. I think this is the right time to make certain that all those questions are addressed.

I. Helsper (Utrecht, NL): Mr. Arnoldussen, we got a bit confused when you were discussing the class D and open systems, because you referred to open systems as making needle punctures or a connection. Were you referring to the sterile connection device kind of connection?

S. Arnoldussen (Ouderkerk a/d IJssel, NL): If you validate the sterile connection device in making the connections and the validation results are all right, then you get a closed system. So, there are no requirements for environmental control then. As to the open system, there are two kinds of open systems, that is the industrial scale system which is a real open system where you need a sterile environment: A grade A, B or C, and there is a system in between a closed and a real open system. That is mentioned in the GMP guidelines for blood banks, the system where you puncture blood bags. So, there is a slight risk of contamination and that should be done in a class D grade area.

I. Helsper: There is also a slight risk with a sterile connection device, because there are conditions to the S of sterile making a connection with the device. I mean what is the degree of air dirtiness acceptable without challenging or jeopardizing the S of the SCD?

S. Arnoldussen: That is what you have to validate and have to prove that the system works well and stays sterile under the conditions you work on. In one of the guidelines it is mentioned specifically, that if you have validated your sterile connection device (SCD) then it could be regarded as a closed system.

I. Helsper: So, if you did not validate, a guideline could be to put it in a class D situation?

S. Arnoldussen: Yes I think so.

IV. Good Clinical Practice (CGP)

GOOD CLINICAL (RESEARCH) PRACTICE

F. Wells

Introduction

The Association of the British Pharmaceutical Industry (ABPI) originally published its guidelines on Good Clinical (Research) Practice (GCP) in 1988. It has subsequently considered at length whether a revision of these guidelines was needed in view of the existence of GCP guidelines endorsed by the European Commission. The decision was taken not to re-issue ABPI guidelines, but this paper is based on the redraft which would have published had we decided to go ahead.

One important aspect considered by the ABPI should be emphasized. It is essential to define "sponsorship" with particular reference to those studies initiated by investigators without direct reference to a pharmaceutical company other than seeking support. In those circumstances, where the company has no wish to include the trial in its own research program, it is reasonable to expect the investigator to assume the role of sponsor as well, and the EC GCP guidelines state that when an investigator independently initiates and takes full responsibility for a trial, the investigator assumes the role of the sponsor as well. The ABPI therefore recommended that whenever a company is sponsoring a clinical trial this should be conducted to GCP standards; that investigators must be expected to assume the role of sponsor in the circumstances defined in the CPMP guidelines; and that investigators should conduct all clinical research projects to GCP standards. A simple guide to GCP, intended for investigators and their colleagues, was published by the Association in September 1992 to facilitate this recommendation.

With regard to audit and inspection, the Association strongly recommended that companies should have internally audited and agreed procedures in place, defined in written Standard Operating Procedures (SOPs).

The protocol

Every clinical trial must have a written and signed protocol. Each clinical protocol must be complete and comprehensive, containing details of the aims of the study, the rationale for the study design and the procedure leading to selection, exclusion, participation and withdrawal of each subject. References should be given when discussing the background to the study. The protocol and all its appendices, together with the case record forms, should contain all the written documentation required by the investigator and his colleagues to conduct the study. While protocols may differ according to the objectives of the study, the overall structure is the same; this is regardless of the phase of the study.

The following principles apply:

- The protocol must define clearly the objectives of the study.
- The protol must be designed to enable the objectives of the study to be met.
- The study must be ethical.
- Adequate measures should be included to determine the safety of the investigational medicine (blood component or plasma derivative).
- The study design must be practical and acceptable for the investigator.
- The protocol must meet all legal/regulatory requirements.

Protocol checklist

– *Standard cover page(s) information:* Formats vary, but standard information should include the following: Protocol title, date of protocol and space for recording amendments, protocol number, phase of study (I-IV), test medicine (name, form, strength), comparator medicines, regulatory status, name of sponsor, name, address and telephone number of monitor, name of principal investigator and associates, signatures of approval of investigator and sponsor.

– *Objectives of the study:* Both primary and secondary objectives must be clearly stated.

– *Rationale of the study:* Description of the medicine, mode of action, and a statement on toxicology/safety aspects.

– *Subject selection:* Number of subjects to be studied, sex, age range, selection, rejection, inclusion and exclusion criteria, and minima and maxima per center for multi-center trials.

– *Study design:* Should state, for example, single or double blinding, control methods (within or between subjects), use of placebo, statistical methods to be used and power calculation, quality control arrangements, and, in the case of a blinded trial, the conditions under which the code may/must be broken, with information on where the trial code will be kept.

– *Ethical and indemnity issues:* The method of obtaining ethical approval, procedures for keeping patient lists, and consideration of confidentiality problems, indemnity and compensation arrangements.

– *Medicine treatment plan:* Form and strength of dose, times of administration, route, duration of treatment, concomitant medicines, number of doses per container, labelling, storage conditions, return of medicines, measures to ensure safe handling, times and periods of effects recording.

– *Parameters to be measured:* For entry into the study, for efficacy, for safety, and for compliance; methods of computation and calculation of effects. (The study parameters should be sufficiently sensitive to measure the putative effects of the medicine under investigation).

– *Time schedule for the study:* The time allocated for the investigator, and for the study as a whole, with the justification for this time schedule.

– *Complications of treatments:* Provisions for dealing with complications of treatments, should they arise.

– *Reporting of adverse events:* Procedures to be adopted for the reporting of adverse events, including by whom, to whom, and how fast.

– *Withdrawals and drop-outs:* A description of how withdrawals and drop-outs should be handled.

– *Follow-up procedures:* Follow-up procedures to be adopted. The protocol should define the end point of the study.

– *Continuation supplies:* The policy regarding continuation supplies, if appropriate, should be specified, and be clear to both investigators and patient subjects.

– *References:* All procedures should be referenced, either in the text or detailed in an appendix.

Selection of investigators and centers

It is the responsibility of the sponsor to inform the investigator of the chemical/pharmaceutical, toxicological, pharmacological and clinical information which should be adequate to justify the nature, scale and duration of the trial as a prerequisite to planning the trial. All relevant information must be included in an Investigator's Brochure.

The invitation to participate in a clinical trial should be extended to the potential investigator by the pharmaceutical physician in charge of the study, or by the medical director. This invitation will emphasize that it is subject to certain conditions being fulfilled, including a satisfactory report from the designated study monitor following a pre-trial inspection of the site.

The following issues should be considered in the selection of investigators and centers, and should be raised during one or more pre-study visits, details of which should be adequately documented and appropriately shared with investigators.

The investigator

As suitable investigator will have appropriate qualifications and experience and sufficient time to devote to the study, and be familiar with the demands a study places upon his resources. The personal integrity and welfare of trial subjects is the ultimate responsibility of the investigator in relation to the trial.

It should be checked whether the investigator is currently running other studies which might make a demand upon his time, energy, subjects and material resources. The investigator and his staff must have sufficient time to conduct the study. If the investigator appears to be disorganized and rushed, questions should be raised about scheduling, staff, and the management of time. Over extended or disorganized clinicians may have little time to fill out case report forms, to keep records, to return telephone calls or to discuss the study. The company should ensure that the investigator is able to fulfil the requirements of the study.

The facilities

A suitable investigator will have adequate facilities including equipment, space, access to laboratories and sufficient staff to support the research to good clinical and laboratory practice standards. Staff will include appropriate medical, clerical, nursing and technical staff. If appropriate, fully functional resuscitation equipment should be immediately available in case of emergency. The personal availability of the investigator should be explored. The adequacy of the resources available should be assessed against the protocol.

The study population

Investigators should have an adequate subject population with the specific illness under study. It may be necessary to obtain the cooperation of other physicians to obtain the sufficient number of subjects. In order to establish a realistic time-table it may be useful to review retrospectively, or prospectively, subjects' notes over, for example, an eight week period to identify those subjects who would have qualified for the study. The investigator would check whether the subjects so identified: a) were a hospital or clinics for the required duration of the study; b) would meet all inclusion/exclusion criteria; c) could have been managed in a manner compatible with the proposed protocol. Such a review would also assist in confirming the suitability of the proposed center.

Multi-center studies

Special provisions should be made for multi-center studies. One investigator may be selected to act as a coordinator. Provision should therefore be made to ensure adequate liaison with the investigators through the coordinator.

Case report form design

The Case Report Form (CRF) must reflect the protocol and provide for the collection of appropriate demographic and historical data for the subject and recording of efficacy and safety data. The accuracy and completeness of clinical trial data collected are heavily dependant on the preparation of appropriate case report forms and alternative electronic methods of data capture, which should aim at both ease of recording and ease of analysis. NCR paper may be used.

The CRF should contain provisions for signature by the investigator as a correct record when the subject has finished the study.

Units of measurement must always be stated and transformation of units must always be indicated and documented.

A copy of the definitive CRF should be retained with the protocol master copy, and a copy should be left with the investigator at the end of the study for archiving purposes.

The investigator should always make a confidential record to allow the unambiguous identification of each patient.

For electronic data processing, SOPs for the handling systems must be in place, and only authorized persons should be able to enter or modify data in the computer, and there should be a record of changes and deletions.
Such systems should be designed to allow correction after loading, and the correction must appear in an audit file. The sponsor must ensure the greatest possible accuracy when transforming data. The sponsor must maintain a list of persons authorized to make corrections and protect access to the data by appropriate security systems.

Ethical approval

In 1964 the 18th World Medical Assembly, meeting in Finland, adopted the Declaration of Helsinki on recommendations guiding medical doctors in biomedical research involving human subjects. This was revised at subsequent World Medical Assemblies – Tokyo in 1975, Venice in 1973 and Hong Kong in 1989. The current revision of the Declaration of Helsinki appears as Appendix III. It is the accepted base for clinical research ethics and must be known, understood and followed by all persons involved in the conduct of clinical trials.

All protocols for clinical trials should be reviewed and approved by a properly constituted independent research ethics committee. The objectives of such committees are to protect subjects of research, to preserve their rights, and to provide public reassurance. Guidelines on the constitution and methods of working of such research ethics committees were issued by the Royal College of Physicians in September 1984, and the UK Department of Health issued a document covering the same subject in 1991. The Department of Health recommends the setting up of Local Research Ethics Committees (LRECs) on a district or unit basis as appropriate. Their constitution must include medical and non-medical members, and the lay public must always be represented. The list of members present during each approval should be given. No investigator should participate in the approval process of a clinical trial in which he or she is involved. One specific responsibility of an LREC is approval of the investigator.

The protocol for a multi-center trial may appropriately be reviewed and approved (on behalf of all committees which would otherwise individually be required to consider the protocol) by a central or a nominated LREC. An example of a LREC is likely to command the confidence of LRECs is that established by the Royal College of General Practitioners.

Research ethic committees must satisfy themselves regarding the protocol, consent procedures (see section Informed consent), documentation, adequacy of confidentiality safeguards, payments to investigators and to subjects, and the existence of satisfactory indemnity and compensation arrangements. LRECs must satisfy themselves regarding the experience, qualifications, and availability of the investigator, other local facilities, and the availability of eligible trial subjects. Research ethics committees should review protocol amendments, subject information sheets, and extensions of protocols, and should receive details of serious adverse events arising during the course of a trial which they have approved. A copy of the approval should be received by the sponsor before the trial begins, and held thereafter for archival purposes.

The investigator must inform the ethics committee when the trial has finished. The opinion of the ethics committee must be sought if re-evaluation of the ethics of the trial appears to be called for.

Informed consent

The purpose of informed consent is to ensure that the person who is a subject for human experimentation of any form is made fully aware of that experimentation and his/her own rights and responsibilities within that experiment. Subjects should be made aware of the purpose of the trial and of known benefits and risks. Freely given informed consent protects the subject, the investigator and the sponsor. Subjects should be provided with pertinent information in both oral and written form whenever possible, and be able to volunteer without pressure to participate. They should also be given every opportunity to ask questions about their involvement in the trial. They should be free to withdraw from the trial at any stage and without reason. They should understand that subjects cannot be recruited into a trial until they have given this consent.

Informed consent should be written, signed and dated by the person receiving the information, and the investigator or the person designated to obtain consent. If, in exceptional circumstances, it is not possible to obtain written consent, there should be a statement in the CRF, with the investigator's signature that verbal consent has been given. If possible, an independent witness should verify oral consent on the consent form. For non-patient volunteers, consent must be written. Written consent should be obtained only after an explanation of the study, its aims, the comparator treatments (including placebo), benefits and risks and, where appropriate, an explanation of alternative standard recognized medical therapy has been given. It may be preferable to obtain the signature of a witness to the fact that the subject comprehends what is involved and has been given the opportunity to ask questions. If so, this should be recorded. Information must only be provided to the subject by an individual who is thoroughly familiar with the trial product and the protocol.

Subjects enroled in a trial should be provided with a card bearing information identifying that he/she is in this trial. This should also be stated in the medical records.

In studies on subjects who are unable to give consent for any reason such as unconscious patients or those with severe mental illness or handicap, consent in writing should be obtained from the spouse, parent, guardian or other close relative. As detailed in the Declaration of Helsinki, when a minor is able to give consent, this should be obtained in addition to the consent of the minor's legal guardian (appendix III). A subject consent form is dependant on the type and complexity of the study. The signed consent form must be kept in the subject's study file at the investigator site. The subject and/or legal representative must also be provided with a copy of the signed form. Informed consent must be obtained prior to a subject entering a study.

Contact addresses and telephone numbers should be given in case action is needed at another place. This should be such that response can be given within an hour.

The elements of informed consent

The elements of informed consent are dependent upon the complexity of the study, nature of the compound under investigation, and its stage of development. The nature and scope of the informed consent should be part of the review procedure carried out by the ethics committee reviewing the study. The subject should be told of the following aspects:

- The study is a research procedure, the nature and type of which will be explained.
- The scope, aims, purpose and duration of the research are usually described together with known benefits (if any) of participating in the study, and known and foreseeable risks and discomforts the subject might experience on participating in the study.
- Appropriate alternative recognized standard therapies or procedures should be disclosed so that the individual can determine whether or not he/she wishes to participate in the study.
- That his/her participation in the study is confidential, but the subject should be made aware that this participation will be disclosed to his/her general practitioner and may be disclosed to a regulatory authority.
- That personal information may be scrutinized during inspection by competent authorities and/or authorized persons, but that this will be treated as strictly confidential and not be publicly available.
- Any compensation plan available will be explained to the subject should he/she be injured by participating in the study. For volunteers, reference should be made to the 1988 ABPI Guidelines for Medicinal Experiments in Non patient Human Volunteers. For patients, reference should additionally be made to the 1991 ABPI Guidelines on Compensation for Drug Induced Injury.
- The name and telephone number of the appropriate contact points should be given to the subject in case they are needed whilst participating in the study.
- An emphatic statement that participation is entirely voluntary.
- Statements laying out the circumstances under which the subject's participation in the study would be terminated.
- The fact that he/she has a right to withdraw from the study at any time without prejudice or justification, and without any jeopardy to the subsequent care to the subject. If the patient withdraws because of any adverse event, however, the reason should be given.

- Disclosure of any medicines (or alcohol) currently being taken is required. Subsequently, the subject should be required to inform the investigator of any changes in other drug use occurring during the study. The possibility of drug dependence of the subject must be checked.
- Disclosure of any new findings which adversely affect the safety of the subject which may become available on the compound under investigation during participation in the study.
- The approximate number of other people participating in the particular study.
- The consent form will contain a statement to the effect the subject has understood the explanation given by the clinician. It must be signed by the subject and preferably by a witness to the explanation who is unconnected with the trial. The subject should be allowed to keep the written explanation for future reference. Copies of the informed consent form should be kept by the company and by the investigator. The Data Protection Act and the Access to Medical Records Act must be borne in mind.
- The information must be presented in a language that is understandable to the subject and/or his representative.
- Adequate time should be allowed for the subject to decide whether he/she wishes to participate in the study.
- Consent must always be given in writing by the subject in a non-therapeutic study, where there is no direct clinical benefit to the subject.

Subjects incapable of giving personal consent

- If the subject is incapable of giving personal consent the inclusion of such patients may be acceptable if the ethics committee is in principle in agreement, and if the investigator is of the opinion that participation will promote the welfare and interest of the subject. The agreement of a legally valid representative that participation will promote the welfare and interest of the subject should also be recorded by a dated signature.

Monitoring of clinical studies

Responsibilities of study monitors

the activities of designated study monitors should be clearly set out and governed by good quality SOPs. The main responsibility of the designated study monitor is to oversee the progress of the study and to ensure that it is conducted and reported in accordance with the protocol. The study monitor should be adequately qualified and trained and be fully cognisant of the drug under investigation and the protocol and its requirements. The monitor may be either medically and/or scientifically qualified.

Monitoring is normally conducted by on-site visits to the investigator at regular intervals (i.e. 4-6 weeks) to determine study progress and protocol compliance, to check and retrieve case report forms and to check trial supplies. On-site monitoring may be supplemented by telephone calls of which a written record should be kept, and by written communications. Full records, including telephone contact reports, visit reports and copies of follow-up letters should be carefully maintained by the monitor. Monitors should ensure that they or some other responsible and appropriate company person(s) are available to the investigator at any time for consultation or for the reporting of suspected adverse drug reactions. They should also ensure that a mechanism exists to enable an appropriate responsible person to be informed of the nature of blinded clinical trial material within one hour in an emergency.

Pre-trial visit(s)

The purpose of the pre-trial visit is to check and record general and specific aspects of the trial. These may include:

- Assessment of the investigator's experience and competence in trials.
- By discussing each section of the protocol with the investigator, and with his staff in detail, assessment of the feasibility of the protocol requirements in that unit (including adequate staff space, facilities and equipment), confirmation of the investigator's understanding of the drug and the nature of the study, and his/her understanding of his/her obligations in undertaking the study – including involvement in investigator meetings and coping with data resolution.
- Discussions with other staff associated with the trial including nursing staff, technicians and pharmacists.
- Confirmation of procedures such as adverse event reporting, financial agreement, study agreement, confidentiality agreement, time intervals, target dates and publication plans.
- Confirmation that regulatory requirements, research ethics committee procedures, and informed consent procedures will be met.
- Explanation of procedures regarding the safe keeping and storage of drug supplies, trial code and of breaking the code under the conditions described in the protocol.
- Assessment of the unit's ability to undertake data analysis where applicable.
- Discussions to ensure acceptance and availability of all necessary documents.

Immediately prior to the proposed starting date, it may be advisable to visit the units to ensure that the investigator has the final protocol, all the required materials, CRFs, drug supplies, subject information leaflets and diaries as appropriate, in order to initiate the study formally.

Relevant details should be recorded and a copy may be provided to the investigator.

Laboratory and clinical measurements

The study monitor should consider a number of aspects, when discussing the study with the investigator. These should include an assessment made at the pre-monitoring visit, with a record of the facilities available and of the competence and experience of the proposed unit, investigator and his staff to undertake the measurements defined in the protocol.

– *Laboratory measurements:*

– Laboratory methods of assay and laboratory normal values should be obtained at a pre-trial visit. In long-term trials it may be necessary to obtain laboratory normal values at the end of the study for comparison. It is relevant to review the laboratory's quality control procedures and data, including calibration of equipment and validation of computer systems. The monitor must be informed if laboratory methods or normal values are changed.
– In multi-center trials, investigations should be undertaken at a central location, equipped to handle volume, wherever possible to avoid inter-laboratory variations. If this is not feasible, there may need to be standardization and checking against reference samples.
– Consideration should be given to random checking of appropriate measurements, for example standard reference samples during drug assays. Laboratory methods (good laboratory practice) whether in house or on contract should be detailed. The presence or absence of a Good Laboratory Practice (GLP) certificate should be noted.
– Details should be given on how blood samples should be obtained, stored, transported and analyzed.
– Consideration should be given to how records are stored, and to whether a back-up procedure is in place for emergencies.
– References to methods should be quoted and updated as necessary.

– *Clinical measurements:*

– Variations in methods and standards between investigators in a multi-center study should be minimized as far as possible.
– Investigational measurements should be accurately defined in the protocol. These include, for example, blood pressure lying (after x minutes), diastolic (phase IV or V), ECG (full twelve lead or rhythm strip), serum calcium fasting (with or without compression).
– Procedures should be defined to ensure full subject comprehension for any tests in which lack of understanding could influence results. These include, for example, visual analogue scales and glucose monitoring.
– All procedures should be referenced, either in the text or detailed in an appendix.
– Published references to methods should be quoted whenever possible.

Monitoring visits during the study period

Regular visits should be made to all trial centers during the study period. The frequency of these visits must depend upon the nature of the study and shall be agreed in principal in advance.

An in-house record should be kept and a copy sent to the investigator. Copies should be kept of any follow-up letters sent to the investigator.

The monitoring visit should normally include:

– Assessment of overall progress of the study including the investigator's and his staff's active participation and the continuing ability of the center to participate in the study.

- Determination of the recruitment status since the last visit, ensuring that informed consent has been obtained for all subjects, the number of withdrawals or drop outs and the reasons, and the situation regarding adverse events. It is the responsibility of the sponsor to consider promptly, jointly with the investigator, all serious adverse events and take appropriate measures necessary to safeguard trial subjects, and to report to the appropriate authorities according to their requirements.
- Collection of CRFs. It is absolutely essential that these are checked with the investigator for a preliminary assessment of the completeness, legibility, adherence to the protocol, particularly inclusion/exclusion criteria, signatures, aberrant values and other factors. CRFs should be compared against the original notes. If corrections are made on CRFs, they should be dated, and initialled by the investigator, and should not obscure the original entry.
- Checking medicines supply records. This may involve visiting the pharmacist to check the drug dispensing logs and to ensure sufficient medicine supplies to allow uninterrupted progress of the study including checking expiry dates of batches in stock and checking storage conditions of trial supplies.
- Checking storage of sealed envelopes and/or masked allocation schedules, and the "unblinding" documentation.
- Collection, where appropriate, of unused or returned drugs.
- Collection, where appropriate, of samples for analysis.
- In addition to checking CRFs, any other raw data such as Holter tapes and photographs should be checked for correct labelling, dating and signatures.
- Completion and documentation of all laboratory investigations.
- Laboratory values outside a clinically accepted reference range or values that differ importantly from previous values must be evaluated, and commented on by the investigator.
- Checking, where appropriate, any special test equipment, including documentation of calibration and performance.
- Ascertaining any problems which have arisen or are foreseen.

Following the visit and collections of CRFs the forms should be reviewed and any recommendations which might arise should be recorded by the monitor for change and authorization, on the CRF, by the investigator (as in Collection of CRFs above).

The monitor must ensure that the investigator is kept fully informed of all matters relating to the study which could impinge on the safety or ethics of the study.

Monitor's responsibilities after clinical completion of the study

The study monitor should:

- Ensure that all documentation is complete, including laboratory investigations.
- Ensure collection and safe keeping of all relevant records in accordance with company policies and regulatory requirements.

- Ensure collection or destruction of all unused medicines supplies and an appropriate record kept, to facilitate subsequent audit.
- Ensure collection of all code break envelopes recording any which have been opened, and the reasons for so doing.
- Ensure the compilation of the final report (either by the investigator, in house or both). If the report is written by the sponsoring company, it should be countersigned by the investigator. It should include confirmation of compliance with GCP.
- Ensure that the protocol and all documentation relating to the trial is retained by the sponsor in the trial master file.
- Check that the investigator has made arrangements to archive the files.

Investigator agreements

The work performed by the investigator on behalf of the pharmaceutical company should be the subject of a formal agreement, including financial arrangements where appropriate, respected by both sides.

The principal clinical investigator will be a medical or dental practitioner selected by the company to conduct a particular study.

Investigator responsibilities

The investigator must:

- Submit an up-to-date curriculum vitae to the sponsor, and, if necessary, to the relevant authorities.
- Ensure that he/she is fully familiar with the properties of the investigational medicinal product(s), as described in the Investigator's Brochure.
- Ensure that he/she has sufficient time to conduct and complete the trial, nominating if appropriate a local study coordinator to assist in the administration of the trial.
- Ensure that he/she has adequate support staff and appropriate facilities (including laboratories and archive space) which are available for the duration of the trial.
- Ensure that other trials do not divert essential subjects or facilities away from the trial in hand.
- Agree a publication policy with the sponsor before the start of the study.
- Obtain local research ethics committee approval, and, if necessary, approval of the unit management, and provide details of the ethics committee membership and working procedures to the sponsor, before the study commences.
- Provide retrospective data on numbers of patients who would have satisfied the proposed entry criteria during proceeding time periods, in order to assure a realistic but adequate requirement rate for the trial.
- Agree and sign the protocol submitted to the ethics committee.

- Agree to work to this protocol, and accept that no changes should be made to the protocol without agreeing them with the sponsor, except if necessary to eliminate an apparent immediate hazard to a subject; such changes should form a protocol amendment to be signed by the investigator and the sponsor, and resubmitted by the investigator to obtain further ethics committee approval.
- Obtain informed consent from trial subjects in accordance with the Declaration of Helsinki before including them in the trial, ideally in writing, otherwise witnessed indicating the date, and provide a specimen copy of the consent form to be used, if this has not been provided by the sponsor.
- With the subject's consent inform the family doctor preferably prior to starting the trial.
- Ensure that subjects enroled in a trial are provided with an information sheet giving details about the trial, which should include contact addresses and telephone numbers where further information can be obtained in case of action needed at another place.
- Provide relevant information about the subject, in addition to other details provided by the sponsor, to all staff members involved with the trial or with other elements of the management of the subject, whilst ensuring that the confidentiality of all identifiable information about the subject is respected by all persons involved.
- Ensure that deliveries of investigational medicinal products from the sponsor are correctly received by a responsible person, such as a pharmacist, and are recorded.
- Ensure that investigational products are handled and stored safely and properly and are only dispensed to trial subjects in accordance with the protocol.
- Ensure that any unused products are returned to the sponsor, or other disposal as agreed in the protocol.
- Conduct the trial properly so that it is possible to reconcile the medication delivery records with records of usage and of return of unused stock when the trial is completed, giving account for any discrepancies, and signing certificates of delivery and of returns, and/or destruction.
- Ensure that the trial randomization code envelopes are kept safely, and that they are returned intact to the sponsor, if not used, at the end of the study; the treatment code should only be broken in accordance with the protocol, and the sponsor should be consulted or informed whenever this is done, with reasons.
- Ensure that the data and CRFs are complete and accurate, and are completed in accordance with the protocol, with any corrections to data (which must be dated and initialled) are made in such a way so as not to obscure the original entry.
- Make available the data (CRFs) results and interpretations of the trial to the sponsor.
- Maintain for as long as required all patient files and other source data relating to the study, including copies of case record forms. For example, patient identification codes are required by the EC directive to be kept for 15 years.

- Ensure that subjects are told about any information which becomes available during the trial which may be of relevance for them.
- Notify the sponsor (and if applicable the local research ethics committee, and the relevant authorities) immediately of any serious adverse events, irrespective of (apparent) causality, with appropriate documentation.
- Agree with, and sign, the final report of the trial; for multi-center trials the signature of the coordinating investigator may suffice if this is stated in the protocol.
- Maintain an accurate set of clinical records, which should clearly and prominently indicate that the subject is taking part in a clinical trial; this is to provide essential source material for auditing purposes, making these available (whilst still maintaining requisite confidentiality of personal subject details) at any stage during the trial to the monitor or quality assurance personnel from the sponsor company and/or relevant authorities for verification/audit/inspection purposes.
- Maintain confidentiality of the information provided by the sponsor.
- Must ensure appropriate medical care/follow up of trail subjects after the trial.

Reports of studies

A report must be written for every study. This report should present the results of trials accurately, clearly, unambiguously, without bias and should provide a balanced and reasonable interpretation of the data. It may also be used as the basis for a publication in a medical journal.

Some investigators have data handling facilities and statistical expertise at their disposal. However, it is essential to ensure that whatever analyses and facilities are used fulfil GCP standards.

Companies should also require that company pharmaceutical physicians, and their staff, prepare internal company reports of clinical trials which should be signed off. Such reports should follow this suggested format:

Introduction
- Background to the study, importance of condition being treated, frequency, severity, sequelae and mortality.
- Previous work with other related drugs.
- Previous work (pre-clinical/clinical) with test drug.
- Objectives of the study.

Methods
- Investigational centers.
- Research ethics committee approval.
- Subject selection.
- Nature of study (blind, crossover, etc.).
- Treatments: types, dosage, frequency and duration, and allocation.

- Measurements.
- Data handling procedures.
- Statistical methods.

Results
- Subject demography.
- Efficacy and safety data analyses.
- Deviations from the study plan or protocol (described and justified).

Discussion

Conclusions

References

Appendices

These appendices may include:
- Curriculum vitae of each principal investigator.
- Listing of individual subject demographic parameters.
- Listing of individual subject efficacy parameters
- Listing of individual subject safety parameters.
- Batch numbers of materials used.
- Audit report.
- Any other relevant data.

Individual study reports must be signed off by the investigator and appropriate company staff.

The sponsor should retain the final report for five years beyond the lifetime of the product, and all other documentation for the lifetime of the product.

Statistics

The sponsor must use validated, error-free, data processing programs with adequate user documentation. Appropriate measures should be taken by the monitor to avoid overlooking missing data or including logical inconsistencies.

The following aspects of statistics should be considered:
- Proper statistical consideration should be given in the design of studies to the elimination of bias.
- The study protocol should be reviewed during its design by a statistician.
- The statistician must ensure the integrity of the data during their processing.
- Consideration should be given to the "power" of the study in terms of the likelihood of detecting meaningful treatment differences. Studies with insufficient numbers of subjects to provide the required power are unethical as is the entry or inclusion of excessive numbers of subjects.

- The general type and scope of statistical analyses to be used should be specified in the protocol. Analysis of the study should be either conducted by or reviewed by the statistician. Planned interim analyses should be specified in the protocol.
- An account should be taken of both missing and unused data points during statistical analysis. All omissions of this type should be documented to enable review by an outside agency. Data points involving adverse reactions should, however, never be omitted from the final report. If a computer assigns missing values automatically, this should be made clear.

Supplies for clinical trials

Test drugs, active standard control drugs, and placebos used in blinded randomized trials should, wherever possible, be indistinguishable by appearance, taste, smell and other physical characteristics. If changes are made to the control drug formulation, then an in vitro comparative study should be done. Consideration should also be given to the need for an in vivo bioavailability study.

Supplies for new test compounds for clinical trials must be labelled to comply with the Medicines (Labelling) Regulations 1976 (SI No 1726), and show that supplies are for clinical research purposes. Preparations or at least their containers should carry some unique identification code so that, if found, the nature of the supply and trial concerned can be quickly identified and a suitable contact point used for advice. The container should include information to enable an appropriate responsible person to be informed of the nature of blinded clinical trial material within one hour in an emergency (see Responsibilities of study monitors).

Wherever possible, supplies should be made available in packages suitable for issue to the subject (preferably in a child-proof container) rather than requiring dispensing from bulk container. Clinical trial material should be stored in a locked place, at controlled temperature and humidity if possible.

Investigators should be supplied under sealed cover with a key to the coding of the drugs in double-blind studies so that, should an emergency arise, it is possible to identify the actual treatment an individual subject is receiving without delay. It is essential to use systems whereby the treatment code for an individual subject can be broken without the identity of treatments for all other subjects in the study becoming known.

It is the responsibility of the investigator to establish a system regarding investigational medicinal products to ensure that deliveries from the sponsor are correctly received by a responsible person, usually a pharmacist; that such deliveries are recorded; certificates of delivery and returns must be signed.

Accountability by investigators for materials used in clinical trials is required as an indicator of good clinical research practice (GCP). Such procedures increase confidence in the correct dosages being prescribed and, if unconsumed drugs are returned, provide information about subject compliance. This also helps to prevent investigators treating named subjects with test drugs in an unauthorized manner outside the trial protocol.

If the protocol has determined that continuation supplies are appropriate (See Continuation supplies), companies should ensure that for medicines supplied in this way the investigator understands where any liability may fall.

Clinical trial supplies (particularly biological preparations) should be re-assayed during, and at the end of, a clinical trial if there are any concerns about suitability of a preparation under field conditions.

Sufficient samples of each batch and a record of its analyses and characteristics must be kept for reference.

Contact addresses and telephone numbers should be given in case action is needed at another place. This should be such that response to a request for unblinding by a responsible person can be given within an hour.

Quality Assurance

Trials should be subjected to an independent quality assurance procedures especially those destined for regulatory use. This function should be undertaken by personnel who are functionally independent from those conducting the study. All methods of data capture, whether electronic or manual, should be subject to validation. Additionally, all electronic systems should also be subject to validation.

The quality assurance personnel may carry out some or all of the following functions:

Pre-study auditing

- Ensure the appropriate regulatory certificate is obtained.
- Ensure that the protocol is in accordance with appropriate legal and ethical requirements, with research ethics committee approval and agreement to adhere to the Declaration of Helsinki.

During study auditing

- Random inspection of work procedures relevant to clinical studies which can reasonably be inspected by an external auditor within the ethical/legal considerations of human investigations, such as timing of blood samples.
- Inspection of the ongoing progress of the study (documentation and CRFs) especially the systems and study monitoring and drug accountability in order to ensure that the study is being conducted to the appropriate guidelines and/or regulations. Records need to be kept of the audit.

Post-study auditing

- Conduct appropriate reviews and audit of study reports to ensure that they properly describe the methods used and that the results accurately reflect the raw data.
- Written reports of audits should be provided to the appropriate functional groups.

Inspection by competent authorities

- Sites, facilities, laboratories, data and documentation, must also be available for inspection by the competent authorities.

Archiving

Notwithstanding existing regulations, investigators should retain copies of all records pertaining to the study for at least 15 years from the end of the study, and sponsors should retain the trial master file for the lifetime of the product.

The secure place (archive) shall have controlled access and be managed in such a way as to prevent loss of, or tampering with, the records.

Electronic means of data storage may be used, providing it is validated, and that a back-up mechanism exists. Hard copy may be required, and must therefore be available if necessary.

The following is a list of document types which should be retained by the sponsor for each study in a trial master file, and may include:

- Signed protocol.
- Protocol amendments and extensions.
- Curriculum vitae of each investigator.
- Formal agreement with investigator.
- List of investigators and centers.
- Name and address of principal investigator.
- Declarations that informed consent has been obtained.
- Subject information sheet.
- Indemnity agreement.
- Research ethics committee constitution and membership.
- Research ethics committee review document.
- Regulatory approval.
- Adverse event data.
- Randomization schedule.
- Monitoring visit reports.
- Master case record forms.
- Completed case record forms.
- Test substances documentation.
- Laboratory normal ranges (where applicable).
- Correspondence (letters and telephone call reports).
- Relevant listings, tabulations or statistical reports.
- Audit confirmation.
- Signed final report.

The final report must be retained by the sponsor, or subsequent owner for 5 years beyond the lifetime of the product. Any changes of ownership of the data should be documented.

All data and documents should be made available if requested by relevant authorities.

Conclusion

As in 1988, this document is intended to provide guidance for ABPI member companies on GCP, and has been redrafted to take into consideration both the CPMP and the WHO Guidelines on GCP. It advises on standards for the conduct of all phases of clinical research, and should be understood and acted upon by both industry and academic researchers.

Application of the principles of good clinical research practice as exemplified in this document will be of crucial importance in achieving and maintaining high standards of clinical research which is in the best interest of the pharmaceutical industry, the practising physician and the patient.

Reference

European CPMP Good Clinical Practice Guideline; European Communities Council Directive 91/507, May 1991, Brussels.

ERROR POLICIES AT THE BEDSIDE – QUALITY MANAGEMENT OF BLOOD TRANSFUSION IN DUTCH HOSPITALS

N.S. Klazinga

Introduction

This article explores the nature and effectiveness of quality management activities in the field of blood transfusion in hospitals. The first part of the article describes the position of blood transfusion as a topic for Quality Assurance (QA) in relation to other popular QA items in European hospitals and more in detail, in the context of peer-review committees in Dutch hospitals. A brief overview will be given of the infrastructure of QA in Dutch hospitals and the scope and format of a national program for the development of practice guidelines. The implementation and effect of a national practice guideline on blood transfusion policy in hospitals formulated in 1982 is discussed in detail. Furthermore a synthesis of a series of audit-studies on blood transfusion performed in different hospitals will be provided. The article concludes with a description of the different phases of realizing improvements in blood transfusion practice and the factors influencing the improvement.

Blood transfusion as a topic for quality assurance

Under the aegis of QA a large number of activities are performed in hospitals. As part of a recent concerted action program a total of 276 hospitals in 15 countries were asked about existing committees in their institution [1]. Table 1 gives an overview of the answers provided. Although this group of hospitals is not representative for all European hospitals (the cohort consists of hospitals basically interested to participate in a study on QA and teaching- and university hospitals are over-represented) the percentages provide an indication of the relative attention given to specific topics. A Blood Transfusion Committee seems to be less often functioning than one on hospital infection or drugs policy, however, their existence is comparable to the existence of committees on medical audit, incident reporting and risk management. Table 2 originates from the results of the same study and shows the existence of guidelines on blood transfusion in general and the presence of standard blood ordering lists in specific, related to other topics covered through guidelines. Asked whether the hospital knew (and thus recorded) its transfusion reaction rate as a percentage of the total number of

Table 1. Committees on blood transfusion: COMAC/HSR/QA study 1990-1993.

Hospital infections	79%
Drugs/therapeutics	73%
Medical records	44%
Autopsy meetings	36%
Incident report	25%
Blood transfusion	22%
Medical audit	20%
Risk management	20%

n = 276 hospitals in 15 countries

Table 2. Guidelines on blood transfusion: COMAC/HSR/QA study 1990-1993.

Druguse	68%
Infection control	65%
Record keeping	55%
Preoperative assessment	52%
Blood transfusion	49%
Blood ordering	43%
Bedsores	42%
Autopsy rate known	71%
Infection rate known	35%
Transfusion reaction rate known	52%

n = 276 hospitals in 15 countries

Table 3. Twelve priority topics medical audit: Dutch hospitals 1977-1992.

Pre-operative assessment	30%
Record keeping	20%
Anti-coagulant use	16%
Antibiotics policy	15%
Blood transfusion policy	15%
Reanimation policy	12%
Bladder catheterization	10%
Triage at the emergency ward	9%
Intercollegial consultations	8%
Infusion policy	8%
CITO-tests	7%
Bedsores policy	7%

n = 1084 topics brought forward in 101 prioritye meetings

transfusions, 52 per cent of hospitals answered affirmative compared to 35 per cent that reported to know their post-operative infection rate in clean wound surgery.

Another indication of the popularity of blood transfusion as a topic for QA is provided by Table 3. This table lists the number of times a specific topic was chosen as priority 1, 2 or 3 for medical audit activities in a series of 101 priority meetings held with groups of medical specialists in Dutch hospitals between 1977 and 1992. On this list blood transfusion, together with antibiotics policy, stands on the fourth place.

Table 1, 2 and 3 suggest that, although blood transfusion does not appear to be the highest priority for QA in hospitals, it still is among the more popular themes.

General infrastruture of quality assurance in Dutch hospitals

The past ten years hospital managers and clinicians have realized that a lot of already ongoing activities in their hospitals are in essence part of QA. All activities in which health care is evaluated and criteria and protocols are formulated, are in fact QA. Although the following review is not complete it touches upon most of the QA activities in hospitals identified sofar [2]. One must realize that most hospitals have some, but hardly any have all, of the mentioned QA mechanisms in place. Three levels of QA activities in hospitals can be identified.

Level 1: Direct forms of QA performed daily

This category consists of all activities in which health care providers exchange information and compare the actual clinical situation of the patient with their expectations. Different methods are used to organize patient review and information exchange, but in most hospitals one can find:

- Clinical rounds (systematic review by bed-side visits).
- Visit on paper (review of the patients by means of the medical record).
- Patient transfer meetings (meetings of the medical staff of a department at the beginning and/or the end of the day to discuss all current patients).
- Nursing rounds and nursing patient transfer.
- Multidisciplinary meetings about specific patients.
- Tumour/oncology meetings.
- Record keeping (the medical as well as the nursing record).
- Information exchange about test results.
- Radiology meetings to discuss the results of tests
- Discharge letters to other specialists or general practitioners.

Level 2: Indirect forms of quality assurance performed periodically

This category consists of a large number of committee activities in which either criteria/protocols/standards are developed, or specific elements of the health care process are reviewed.

– *Autopsy meetings:* One of the oldest forms of peer review in which evaluation of health care takes place is based on the results of an autopsy. The findings of the pathologist are compared with the findings of the clinician. Although the number of autopsies seems to decline in most countries, the autopsy meeting is still a vital element of medical evaluation. Apart from case-based review, several hospitals review their deathcauses also on an aggregated level on a yearly basis.

– *Drugs committee:* Drugs committees are installed to formulate guidelines about the use of drugs in the hospital. Most of the times this results in a formularium which mentions the drugs that can be used in the hospital. Drugs committees seem particularly useful in formulating guidelines on antibiotic use.

– *Infection committee:* This committee, often assisted by a hygienist, formulates guidelines for infection prevention and tries to monitor the infections that occur in the hospital. Registration systems for infections are far from uniform.

– *Incident committee:* Hospitals in The Netherlands have formalized procedures for incident reporting. The incident committee is not to judge whether the incident was based on a fault of a practitioner but has to look for ways to prevent incidents in the future.

– *Ethical committees:* These committees are involved in judging the appropriateness of clinical trials in the hospital. In Dutch hospitals it is compulsory to send research proposals to the research ethical committee of the hospital before the research can be executed.

– *Committees for medical audit, nursing audit and peer review:* In these committees professionals review their own work. The method is problem based and aims at the continuous formulation of criteria and evaluation of practice. In The Netherlands peer-review committees have been introduced in the seventies and exist at the moment as committees of the medical staffs of approximately 80 per cent of the hospitals. Nursing audit is also becoming popular and is organized on the level of a specific ward and/or the level of the hospital as a whole.

– *Clinical records committee:* A committee that formulates the criteria and procedures for record keeping.

– *Hospital utilization committee:* A committee that looks systematically at the use of material in the hospital (e.g. disposables and catheter use).

– *Blood transfusion committee:* A committee that sets guidelines for blood transfusion policy (for instance the introduction of a blood ordering list) and evaluates the use of blood and blood products like albumine.

– *Risk management:* The running of special programs in the hospital on the safety of devices and buildings.

– *Complaint handling:* Formal procedures, with possibly a special committee to handle patient complaints. The use of patient surveys is sometimes part of the hospital strategy to become acquainted with the wishes or comments of the patients they treat.

– *Medical staff credentials:* A formalized procedure to check the credentials of every new physician who is coming to work in the hospital.

– *APO (Adverse Patient Occurrences):* A method, originally developed in the USA to monitor on a continuous bases those events that could be used as an indicator of potentially bad quality of care. Examples of such "adverse outcomes" are readmittance to the hospital within two days after discharge, readmittance to the Intensive Care Unit, and death during surgery. The APO systems seems at the moment only in use on an experimental basis.

Level 3: Coordination of quality assurance

The activities mentioned under 1 and 2 are many, and it seems evident that an overall QA policy of a hospital asks for overview and coordination of these activities. This is true for the QA activities of medical care and nursing care, but also for the QA activities of the paramedical groups, supportive services and hotel services of the hospital. Coordination of all these activities is usually weak. The concept of "hospital wide QA" is still emerging and there are few hospitals who identified all QA activities in their institution and were able to place them in a "total QA program" using methods as Total Quality Management (TQM) and Continuous Quality Improvement (CQI).

Guidelines on blood transfusion

Complementary to the QA activities in hospitals, and more specific to the activities in peer-review committees, practice guidelines are formulated at national level. In The Netherlands, Consensus Development Conferences (CDC) are organized by the National Organization for Quality Assurance in Hospitals (CBO) [3]. CBO is an independent organization founded in 1979 by the Medical Specialists' Organization and the Medical Association of Hospital Directors. Its purpose is to stimulate and guide QA activities in hospitals. During the implementation of peer-review activities in hospitals, CBO became aware of the physicians' need for national guidelines concerning a number of medical topics. This led CBO to start a Consensus Development Program (CDP) in 1982. Up to 1993 38 consensus conferences have been held. Over the years the use of blood and blood products has several times been the focus of consensus guidelines. The first guideline, issued in 1982, dealt with blood transfusion policy in hospitals and was revised in 1989. A consensus guideline of platelet transfusion was formulated in 1984 and revised in 1990. A guideline on treatment of hemophilia was formulated in 1985 and a report on the use of fresh frozen plasma was released by the Medical Scientific Council of CBO in 1993. Besides assessment of the scientific literature and the formulation of guidelines with the help of experts during a consensus conference, the importance of the implementation of the conclusions in the daily practice of care must also be recognized. CBO therefore conducted an evaluation of the first consensus guideline on blood transfusion policy to assess the effect of this guideline on daily practice of care and on the QA activities in Dutch hospitals.

The conference in 1982 addressed the topics of blood ordering and transfusion policies in hospitals. Transfusion therapy was considered a costly and frequently applied form of treatment with potential risks and complications. Many hospitals at that time did not have well-defined guidelines for a number of aspects of their transfusion policy. These were the main reasons for the choice of this policy as a topic for consensus development.

A working committee consisting of twelve experts prepared statements concerning good health care delivery with respect to blood transfusion therapy. During the conference on 9 October 1982 the members of this committee gave short presentations and defended the statements before an audience. The conference was attended by 320 participants, mainly internists, directors of blood banks, clinical chemists, surgeons and anesthesiologists. The final consensus text was formulated by the working committee a few weeks after the meeting. This text was composed of the statements agreed upon in the public discussion, together with explanatory remarks. The statements were published in the national medical journal (Nederlands Tijdschrift voor Geneeskunde).

Elements of the blood transfusion policy on which explicit recommendations were made in the consensus text include [4]:

- Identification of the blood samples.
- Double testing of the cross-match technique for missed compatibilities.
- Type and screen strategy and registration of irregular antibodies against red blood cells.
- Use of standardized ordering lists for the use of blood in surgery.
- Proportion of whole blood versus red cell concentrates.
- Quality aspects of red cell concentrates.
- Cross-match/transfusion ratio.
- Indications for use of blood and blood products.
- Administration of blood to the patient.
- Blood transfusion reactions.
- Transfusion committee in hospitals.

Implementation of the guidelines

To evaluate the effect of the guidelines on blood transfusion as formulated in 1982 an evaluation was performed by CBO in 1987 [5-7]. The evaluation was done as a survey combined with interviews and an analysis of peer-review studies. Three years after the conference a questionnaire was filled in by the directors of the Dutch blood banks (n = 22). The annual reports of the blood banks between 1981 and 1986 supplied quantitative data. A structured interview comprising 56 questions was held with a representative sample of heads of hospital hematological laboratories (57 out of 183). After the conference a QA study on blood transfusion policy were to have been known performed in 17 of the 183 Dutch hospitals.

Evaluation of CDC; results

– *Questionnaire sent to 22 directors of blood banks:* Out of the 22 directors, 19 had attended the conference. All but one of them had arranged discussions of the text with the hospitals in their region. Sixteen directors had established guidelines for transfusion policy that were consistent with the consensus text.

– *Interview with 57 heads of hematological laboratories:* All but two of the respondents were aware of the existence of the consensus text and 32 (63%) had attended the meeting. In 36 (66%) of the hospitals, the consensus text was discussed and transfusion policy was modified to some extent. These changes primarily concerned the increased use of red blood cell concentrates, the introduction of the "type and screen" (T/S) strategy, and the installation of a blood transfusion committee. Only eight (5%) hospitals could give a synopsis of data concerning the transfusion reactions.

– *Audit studies:* In 17 hospitals, representing nine per cent of all acute-care hospitals in The Netherlands, a formal QA study was performed after the CDC.

Table 4 shows the elements of the consensus statements that were subject of a peer-review study and also the results of the study. For two of the mentioned topics, i.e., the preservation of blood and policy on outdated blood, no recommendations were made at the conference.

Table 5 gives a summary of the characteristics of the 17 QA studies. In seven studies explicit criteria were formulated in advance and in the other ten the criteria had an implicit character, but both types of criteria were consistent with the consensus text. In two studies data collection failed because of inadequate cooperation in filling in of the forms as requested for these studies. Of the remaining 15 investigations, the results of four show that practice in transfusion policy satisfied the criteria but in the other eleven, changes in physician behaviour or procedures with respect to blood transfusion policy appeared to be necessary. In seven cases a re-evaluation was performed and in four this was done annually. These studies dealt with the cross-match/transfusion ratio, the proportion of the whole blood versus red blood cell concentrates, and policy on outdated blood and blood products. Five studies showed improvement in blood transfusion policy, one study showed no changes and in one case blood transfusion was found to be worse than in the year before.

In summary it can be concluded that the T/S strategy together with the use of a blood ordering list seems to have been implemented in many hospitals. Also the administrative procedures as advised in the 1982 guidelines seem to have been implemented in most laboratories and process control through the use of the cross-match/transfusion ratio seems to become more and more common practice. However the recording of the indication for blood transfusion by clinicians seems still to be a problem and CBO also gets the impression that blood transfusion committees are not functioning well in all Dutch hospitals.

In 1994 the consensus guidelines on blood transfusion will be revised for the second time and it seems clear that especially the last mentioned items need additional attention.

Realizing improvement

The realization of improvements in the field of blood transfusion in hospitals seems to follow the same phases that are prevalent in all quality assurance efforts

Table 4. Overview of 17 quality assurance studies on blood transfusion policy.

Topics	Consensus guidelines	Main results
Identification of blood samples	Each hospital should formulate strict rules for the identification of patients' blood samples	983 samples 280: birth date missing 3: family name missing
Registration of irregular antibodies against red blood cells	The finding of irregular antibodies in a patient's blood should at least be recorded in the following places: – in the records of the blood transfusion laboratory – in the report sent by the laboratory to the specialist – in the medical file – in the letter to the general practitioner after discharge – on the patient's blood group card	78 samples Mentioned on patient's blood group label in 70 cases Not mentioned in medical record in eight cases Mentioned to the general practitioner in only four cases
Use of blood order list	Use of a maximum surgical blood order schedule in combination with a "type and screen" procedure for elective surgery is advocated	Number of cross-match tests reduced from 750 to 500 monthly
Proportion of whole blood versus erythrocyte concentrate used	In all cases requiring transfusion because of a shortage of erythrocytes (anemia, blood loss) red blood cells should be used instead of whole blood	Percentage taken by erythrocyte concentrates 85.3 in 1983; 82.2 in 1984; 87.0 in 1985
Cross-match/transfusion ratio	Efficient use of blood can be promoted by calculation of the cross-match/transfusion ratio	Percentage: 1.68 in 1983; 1.72 in 1984; 1.74 in 1985
Preservation of blood	No consensus guidelines available	48-hour supply available for 96 per cent of all blood groups
Out-dated blood	No consesus guidelines available	Percentages: 5.2 in 1983; 3.7 in 1984; 4.9 in 1985

Table 5. Progress of 17 quality assurance studies in Dutch hospitals along the different steps of the audit-cycle.

Step in the procedure	n	Remarks
Selection of topic	17	
Assessment of criteria	17	Explicit in 7, implicit in 10
Collection of data	15	
Introduction of changes	11	Not necessary in 4
Re-evaluation	7	Improvement in 5

[8]. First the *awareness of the problem* needs to exist in all persons that are supposed to modify their behaviour. The awareness on the risks and problems related to blood transfusion seems highest among the directors of blood banks and heads of hematological laboratories and less high among clinicians. Although the problems related to AIDS have suddenly raised the awareness of clinicians, it remains to be seen if each clinician is actually aware of the infection risks of hepatitis C and B and risks of allergic reactions associated with blood transfusions.

After the phase of awareness the *existence of infrastructural and instrumental mechanisms* to work on QA becomes necessary. These can be found in the existence of blood transfusion committees and/or peer-review committees and guidelines on blood transfusion and blood ordering in Dutch hospitals.

When awareness and mechanisms are no longer a problem the hospital challenges the *realization of actual change*. This implies that resistance to the new modes of behaviour needs to be overcome (i.e. clinicians must be reassured that under the new procedures they will always have the blood in time) and the best way to overcome the resistance is to provide feed-back on the actual practice. After this the fourth phase *lasting change* will be reached. In this phase the new behaviour has become an integral part of practice.

With respect to the attempts to improve the practice of blood transfusion in hospitals, the fourth phase seems to be reached for some of the elements of the 1982 guideline but surely not for all. Strategies to improve aspects as the reporting of indications of blood transfusion need again emphasis but should take the four phases of implementation into account.

During the implementation process different factors seem to have been of importance whether a specific hospital was able to improve its practice or did not come any further than phase one or two. One factor seems to be constituted by the logistics of blood banks and the availability of specific blood products within a certain time limit. A blood bank nearby seems to influence the general attitude towards the need for blood storage and safety feelings related to availability. The reimbursement system is another factor that seems to play a role in choosing the use of blood and blood products as a topic for QA. As blood products are payed for by the volume used, in a period of cost-containment management puts pressure on the clinicians and laboratories to rationalize the use. The direct relation with the costs saved make it an ideal theme for utilization review. The enthusiasm of the head of the laboratory and the ability to establish a good working relationship with clinicians based on mutual respect also seems to play an important role in realizing actual change in the blood transfusion practice. Hospital logistics may also play a role. Especially in the first period when new procedures are introduced, laboratories must prove that the clinicians can trust on the availability of sufficient and adequate blood supply when they deem it necessary. Complementary to the ability of the head of the laboratory to act as a trustworthy "change agent" the real cooperation of the clinicians is needed to get the actual improvements in place.

This listing shows that improving the practice of blood transfusion in hospitals is dependent on a lot of different factors and can not be taken for granted once when a guideline is formulated, no matter the soundness of the guideline. Continuous attention to the implementation is needed and this process should rather be looked upon in years than in months. The improvement of blood transfusion policy in hospitals seems to be taking shape in accordance with the way other QA activities are executed. Therefore it seems advisable to incorporate quality management activities on blood transfusion in the general activities on QA existing in the hospitals.

References

1. Klazinga NS. Quality assurance in hospitals. Concerted Action Programme on Quality Assurance in Hospitals: Multicenter comparative study on different Quality Assurance Strategies and their effect on improvement of care with respect to keeping of patient records, prophylactic antibiotic use in surgery, preoperative assessment, prevention and therapy of bedsores. In: Fracchia GN, Theofilatou M (eds). Health Service Research. IOS Press, Amsterdam, Oxford, Washington DC, Tokyo 1993.
2. Klazinga NS. Implementing Quality Assurance in Health Care, a European Perspective. CBO, Utrecht 1990.
3. Klazinga NS, Casparie AF, van Everdingen JJE. Profile of the Consensus Development Program in The Netherlands: National Organization for Quality Assurance in Hospitals (CB). In: Goodman C, Baratz SR (eds). Improving consensus development for health technology assessment: An international perspective. Institute of Medicine, Washington DC 1990:110-7.
4. Herziening Consensus Bloedtransfusiebeleid in Ziekenhuizen. Utrecht, februari 1989.
5. Van Everdingen JJE, Klazinga NS, Casparie AF. Blood transfusion policy in Dutch hospitals. International Journal of Healthcare Quality Assurance 1988;1:16-9.
6. Van Everdingen JJE, Klazinga NS, Dinkelaar RB, van der Does JA. Het gebruik van pre-operatieve bloedbestellijsten in combinatie met de "type and screen" strategie in Nederlandse ziekenhuizen. Tdschr NVKC 1987;12:270-3.
7. Van Everdingen JJE. Consensusontwikkeling in de geneeskunde. Dissertatie. Bohn, Scheltema & Holkema, Utrecht 1988.
8. Final report Concerted Action Programme on Quality Assurance in Hospitals. CBO, Utrecht 1993 (in press).

CONSENSUS PROTOCOLS FOR SUPPORTIVE HEMOTHERAPY

J.Th.M. de Wolf

Why consensus protocols or guidelines?

There are reasons to become interested in consensus protocols or guidelines for transfusion practice.

First, the great *variability in transfusion practice*. Goodnough et al. [1] demonstrated an impressive variability in the use of blood products in 540 patients undergoing elective coronary bypass surgery at 18 tertiary care hospitals; 68% of the patients received red blood cell concentrate (RBC). There were institutions where only 17% of the patients were transfused whereas in other institutions all patients received RBC; 32% of the patients received plasma, the institutional range was 0-97%; 6/18 institutions transfused > 50% of the patients whereas 9/18 transfused less than 20%. Platelet transfusions showed a similar variation. When patient-related and surgical factors were controlled the RBC transfusion practice remained significantly different among institutions. The transfusion of plasma and platelets seemed often prophylactic and unnecessary. Another example of great variability in transfusion practice is the use of plasma in the academic hospitals in The Netherlands. In 1990 the use per hospital bed ranges from 4.22 to 20.26. Although it is obvious that the lowest level of use is not automatically the right level it raises questions about the justification for the variation, the costs and outcome in the patients.

Second, publications reporting *inappropriate/unnecessary use of blood components*. Goodnough et al. [2] defined as indicators for inappropriate transfusion in patients undergoing elective coronary bypass surgery: The transfusion of RBC for blood loss of less then 15% of the blood volume, transfusion of two or less units of plasma in patients with normal pre-operative clotting times and the transfusion of platelets in patients without pre-operative risk factors for platelet-related bleeding like platelet count less then 150×10^9/l, prolonged bleeding time or aspirin ingestion less then seven days before operation. According to these conservative indicators for inappropriate use of blood components 15% of the RBC, 32% of the plasma and 47% of the platelet transfusions were inappropriate or unnecessary, corresponding with 24% of the total costs of blood components. A recent prospective study of Mozes et al. [3] amongst 560 patients with a preset of 15 explicit criteria for the transfusion of blood or blood components showed that from a total of 1930 transfusions almost 40% was inappropriate. Whole blood and cryoprecipitate were used more appropriate than fresh frozen plasma (FFP), RBC and platelets.

Third, questions about the *health outcomes*, harms and benefits of the use of blood components and their alternatives. Especially these three items led to the interest in guidelines in order to improve the quality of care and patient outcomes, and reduce risks. Besides, it was expected that guidelines could control or even reduce health care costs.

Guidelines in transfusion practice

The Institute of Medicine defined practice guidelines as "systematically developed statements to assist practitioner and patient decisions about appropriate health care for specific clinical circumstances", they are meant to help patients and doctors in making decisions.

In 1977, 1985, 1987 and 1988 the National Institutes of Health (NIH) in the USA published guidelines for the use of albumin, FFP, platelets and perioperative red cell transfusion; in 1988 and 1992 the British Committee for Standards in Haematology published guidelines for transfusion for massive blood loss and FFP. In The Netherlands guidelines were published concerning RBC (1982, updated in 1989) and platelets (1990). We will discuss in more detail the guidelines for the use of FFP from the NIH and its influence on the physician's medical behaviour.

The fear of transmission of infectious diseases, especially of the acquired immunodeficiency syndrome, by plasma products led in 1984 to the Consensus Development Conference held by the NIH on FFP. They concluded that there were only a few specific indications for the use of FFP.

- Replacement of isolated factor deficiencies: When specific component therapy is neither available nor appropriate. As for most factors specific concentrates are available only the very rare factor V and XI deficiency may be considered as an indication.
- The reversal of oral anticoagulant therapy: As for the replacement for factor II, VII, IX and X a safe concentrate (prothrombin complex-SD) is available, the use of plasma is rather exceptional.
- Massive blood transfusion: As there is no evidence that the prophylactic use of plasma decreases the transfusion requirements, only those cases in which documented clotting factor deficiencies (prolonged clotting times) might be responsible for or contribute to a hemorrhagic diathesis justifies the use of plasma.
- Hereditary ATIII deficiency: Although a specific concentrate is available, in certain circumstances , like surgery or delivery, plasma can be used as a source of ATIII.
- Thrombotic thrombocytopenic purpura.

The use of plasma as volume expander or as a nutritional source was not justified by the Conference. The effect of this Consensus Conference was disappointing. In The Netherlands the usage of plasma increased from 1984 (the year of the consensus conference) until 1991 with 101%. In 1989 Mozes et al. [3] reported a 84% inappropriate use of plasma. In 1992 Silver et al. [4] reported their experiences at Hartford Hospital in Connecticut where guidelines for the use of FFP, platelets, RBC, cryo and albumin where proposed by the Transfusion Medicine Committee based on NIH consensus and other publications. The guidelines underwent revision after comments of the medical staff. After a trial period modifications were made again. Following this phase the guidelines were considered as hospital policy. During a prospective concurrent review period 38% of 1564 orders for blood components were appropriate according to the guidelines, 68% of the plasma was inappropriate. Altogether despite a very thorough consensus process more than 50% of the blood ordering was inappropriate. Although a few publications reported a decrease in the use of blood products after introduction of guidelines the overall impression is that many guidelines, not only for the transfusion practice, hardly influence medical behaviour [5-7]. Besides, almost all publications concerning the effect of guidelines for transfusion practice focused on diminishing the use of certain blood products and cost-containment and much less or not on quality or patient outcome.

Guidelines and implementation

The NIH Consensus Development Program has served as a model for the development of practice guidelines in many countries. It integrated aspects of three different decision models: 1) the judicial model, in which scientific evidence presented by experts is heard and weighed by competent impartial judges or juries of peers; 2) the scientific mode, in which experts discuss with their peers about the subject; and 3) the town meeting model, in which all persons involved in the field might express their views.

In the last years much criticism is heard from different sides on the guidelines development. Criticism which could very well function as barriers for implementation. More in general critiques are: Guidelines are meant to diminish variability in medical practice; by that there is a risk of standardizing practice around the average, which is not necessarily the best, and might further interfere with innovation; guidelines are used by judge, insurance company, hospital manager or colleague as golden standard from which deviation would be difficult and must be justified; some belief that professional autonomy or clinical freedom is lost. More fundamental are questions as how solid is the scientific evidence on which the guidelines are funded, to what extend does the guideline improve outcome and in relation with the latter how certain are we that "scientific evidence" must be preferred above "collective sense of the profession"? Eddy distinguishes three main types of practice policies according to the strength of the scientific evidence: Standards, guidelines and options. A policy is considered a standard if the consequences of an intervention are sufficiently well known to permit decisions, and if there is virtually unanimity among patients about the desirability of the intervention. In general, standards must be followed in almost every case. A policy is considered a guideline if the outcomes of the intervention are well enough understood to permit decisions about its proper use, and if it is preferred by an appreciable but not unanimous majority of people. Guidelines should be followed in most cases, but depending on the patient, the setting, and other factors they can be tailored to fit individual needs. Options are neutral with respect to recommending the use of the intervention, there are different practices and little evidence for determining which intervention is most appropriate.

Based on the critiques discussed, the implementation of guidelines might be improved by adjusting the guidelines development process according to the recommendations of the Institute of Medicine, of which validity and reliability/reproducibility are very important parts. The purpose of all medical practice is to maintain or improve the health of patients. Starting point for the guideline should be the effects of the intervention on outcomes that are important for patients. Guidelines are valid if they lead to the projected health and cost outcomes. Every guideline should contain: 1) a statement of the strength of the evidence and the expert judgement behind the guidelines; and 2) estimations of the health and costs outcomes expected from the intervention in question, compared with alternative practice. Relevant health outcomes will consider patient perceptions and preferences. Guidelines are reproducible and reliable if another set of experts produces essentially the same statements, and the guideline is interpreted and applied consistently by practitioners. Finally, increasing our knowledge of factors determining or contributing to changes in behaviour of physicians would be very helpful in improving the implementation of guidelines.

References

Eddy D. A manual for assessing health practices and designing practice policies. The explicit approach. ACP, Philadelphia, Pennsylvania 1992.

Field MJ, Lohr KN (eds). Guidelines for clinical practice: From development to use. National Academy Press, Washington DC 1992.

Kaarsenbrood A. Ontwikkeling van medische richtlijnen: De stand van zaken. In: Consensus in de Geneeskunde 1991;A:5-24.

Institute of Medicine. Consensus Development at the NIH: Improving the program. National Academy Press, Washington DC 1990.

1. Goodnough LT, Johnston MFM, Toy PTCY. The variability of transfusion practice in coronary artery bypass surgery. JAMA 1991;265:86-90.
2. Goodnough LT, Soegiarso RW, Birkmeyer JD, Welch HG. Economic impact of inappropriate blood transfusion in coronary artery bypass graft surgery. Am J Med 1993;94:509-14.
3. Mozes B, Epstein M, Ben-Bassat I, Modan B, Halkin H. Evaluation of the appropriateness of blood and blood product transfusion using preset criteria. Transfusion 1989;29:473-7.
4. Silver H, Tahhan HR, Anderson J, Lachman M. A non-computer-dependent prospective review of blood and blood component utilization. Transfusion 1992;32:260-5.

5. Lomas J, Anderson GM, Domnick-Pierre K, Vayda E, Enkin MW, Hannah WJ. Do practice guidelines guide practice? The effect of a consensus statement on the practice of physicians. N Engl J Med 1989;321:1306-11.
6. Haines A, Feder G. Guidance on guidelines. Writing them is easier than making them work Brit Med J 1992;305:785-6.
7. Delamothe T. Wanted: Guidelines that doctors will follow. Implementation is the problem. Brit Med J 1993;307:218.

HOSPITAL BLOOD TRANSFUSION AUDIT SYSTEMS

A.M. Ali, B. Vander Giessen, M.A. Blajchman

Introduction

Good Manufacturing Practices (GMP) is a relatively new concept for those involved in transfusion medicine. Certainly, in Canada, the licensing of the Canadian Red Cross Society as a manufacturer of biologics has required a rapid paradigm shift on the part of the personnel involved in blood collection and component production. They had to incorporate the new rules and regulations that came with this license into their procedures in order to be in compliance. This, however, represented more than a regulations change; it represented a major cultural change. The fact that the required changes caused difficulties for many within the relatively precise and regimented area of blood collection and component production, indicates the potential degree of difficulty to incorporate GMP into the field of clinical transfusion medicine.

How do good manufacturing practices relate to good clinical practice?

The requirements of GMP to ensure the potency, purity, safety and efficacy of blood products are not entirely applicable to the clinician using blood component therapy in the treatment of their patients. The physician should expect that the potency and purity of the blood product ordered, has been ensured by the manufacturer (the blood center). The efficacy, and to some degree the safety, of their choice of treatment though is controllable and the outcome should be closely monitored.

Physicians tend to believe that they make the best therapeutic choices possible for their patients and are generally hostile to the idea of the quality of their practice being reviewed or audited in any way. The "art" of therapy versus the "science" of the process and the possibility of measurement of either leads to contentious debate. However, in one of our earlier studies we demonstrated that what physicians believe they do and their actual practice, are not necessarily the same. For example, during a retrospective audit of blood products transfused in 16 of the hospitals supplied by our blood center, we sent questionnaires to the physicians in these hospitals asking about their transfusion practices. Hypothetical clinical situations that could involve the transfusion of either red cells, plasma or albumin were developed. One question involving each of the blood products was set in a clinical scenario suitable for internal medicine specialists; another was for the surgical team and a third for obstetricians. Each question was developed so that a transfusion trigger might be determined for each specialty group. All replies were anonymous, but the speciality of the physician and their hospital affiliation was required. One question posed for surgeons, involved the transfusion of red cells pre-operatively to a male who was to have an elective resection for a carcinoma of the colon. The history and presurgical work-up had indicated that the patient was in good physical condition, except for some weight loss and a hemoglobin of 114 g/L. Each surgeon was asked if they would have transfused this man. Those who would not have transfused him were given a series of descending hemoglobin levels and asked at what level they would transfuse. Not surprisingly, 88% of the 174 physicians replying would have transfused the man if his pre-operative hemoglobin had been 94 g/L, but only 5% indicated that they would have transfused this man with a hemoglobin of 114 g/L. However, from our audit of 2,473 red cell transfusion episodes, we found that 391 patients received blood pre-operatively. Ninety four (24%) of these were given to patients undergoing elective surgery and were asymptomatic. The mean hemoglobin for this group of patients was 117 g/L. This illustrates clearly the fact that physicians often do not do what they say they should do. Similar evidence has been reported for indications for patients undergoing elective Caesarian section [1]. Some form of qualitative measurement of clinical practice is therefore needed to ensure good transfusion practice.

The use of audits to measure quality

The aim of monitoring transfusion practice should be to achieve optimum efficacy of such therapy and thus optimum blood component utilization. The more common objectives to realize this aim are summarized in Table 1. There is no single approach that will achieve all of these objectives though various methods of education and auditing have been used. The efficacy of an audit process in realizing any of the objectives depends largely on the timing of the procedure in relation to the transfusion.

Table 1. Objectives of qualitative measurement in transfusion therapy.

– Prevent or reduce inappropriate transfusions
– Determine indications for actual blood product use
– Ascertain emerging trends in transfusion practice
– Evaluation indications of doubtful benefit
– Educate users in appropriate use

Prospective audits

This process usually involves using pre-set criteria that have to be met before staff can issue a blood component from the hospital blood bank. This can occur either by direct consultation with the blood bank/transfusion medicine service director or by incorporating the criteria on the product request form.

Many hospitals have an *informal* pre-transfusion audit process in place for some blood components. For example, when requesting platelets the ordering physician has to contact a member of the transfusion medicine team to explain the rationale for their request before the component is released for the use in a given patient. The acceptance of the rationale however, is often dependent on the judgement of the individual authorizing the release.

Alternatively, there are more *formal* consultation processes, such as that used at the Walter Reed Army Medical Center in Washington, DC, that require clearly defined pre-set criteria to be met [2]. The criteria were developed by the hospital transfusion committee for the use of platelet concentrates. All physicians requesting platelets had to obtain a mandatory pre-transfusion consultation with the transfusion service physician. Platelets were then either issued as ordered, the order was modified, or was denied. During the first ten months of this program 23% of the almost 1000 requests were denied and 31% were substantially modified. This resulted in a 56% reduction in use of platelet concentrates during a time that patient load at that hospital increased 38%. Even more impressive, was the fact that three years after the implementation of this system, only 8% of the requests for platelet concentrates had to be altered or denied; demonstrating the efficacy of this process in modifying transfusion practice.

The use of pre-set criteria on the request form to obtain the reason for the request for transfusion is used in many hospitals. One such example was described in a study from the City Veterans Administration Hospital in Iowa [3]. The criteria selected for albumin transfusion were based on those previously published from a consensus style conference and were reviewed by a surgeon, gastroenterologist and clinical pharmacologist from that institution [4]. These criteria were then incorporated into a request form which had to be completed by the clinician prior to albumin being issued. Although product was never denied, the authors found a drop in inappropriate use of albumin from 41% to 26% of transfusions over the year following the implementation of the program.

Both these forms of pre-transfusion review have the advantage that they can prevent or decrease inappropriate transfusions, thereby decreasing the risks to the patient and reducing the wastage of a limited commodity. It is very important to note, however, that in two of the examples cited, the pre-set criteria were agreed upon by a representative group of physicians in the hospital where they were used [2,4]. A local consensus allows for some modification of criteria to encourage the full support of the practising physicians.

These review methods also act as an educational tool. Although the completion of a request form might lead to erroneous information being provided, to ensure the release of the requested product, the repetitive viewing of acceptable criteria printed on the form may act as a learning tool. With the other method, dialogue with the transfusion service physician allows for the specifics of a case to be discussed and also provides education. Certainly in the reported instances, there was an improvement in transfusion practice.

Immediate post-transfusion audit

This process calls for a review of the transfusion that was given the day before. Shanberge, from William Beaumont Hospital, Royal Oak, MI, described the process they introduced to monitor the use of Fresh Frozen Plasma (FFP) [5]. The hospital transfusion committee issued guidelines for FFP use which were similar to those produced by the NIH Consensus Development Conference [6]. Each day the transfusion service prepared a list of patients who had received FFP during the previous 24 hours. The charts of these patients were reviewed and if the guidelines had not been met, the attending physician was contacted for a "one on one" educational discussion. In addition, the indications for FFP use were discussed at teaching rounds for pathology residents, and hematology fellows. During the first nine months of the study, the number of units transfused was reduced by more than 50% and over the subsequent few months, usage of FFP decreased a further 23%; an indication that many FFP transfusions may previously have been administered inappropriately. The evidence of the success of the daily monitoring and continuing education program was provided by the sustained reduction in the number of units of FFP transfused during the following five years. Despite such efforts, a considerable proportion of FFP units transfused were not of obvious benefit to the recipients; 41% of the units given by the medical service and 46% by the surgical team were deemed inappropriate.

At the 1987 American Association of Blood Banks meeting, Dr. Pearl Toy described the results of a comprehensive retrospective but immediate review process that has been used at the San Francisco General Hospital [7]. Two sets of criteria were developed for the various blood products. One set was for the use of the blood bank technologists who used them to screen all transfusions given within the previous 24 hours, utilizing the available pre and post-transfusion laboratory test results. A second set of criteria were for the use of a transfusion medicine resident who reviewed the charts of recipients not meeting the technologists' criteria. If the transfusion was felt to be inappropriate by the transfusion medicine resident, the blood bank director discussed the case with the physician who ordered the transfusion. The case was also reviewed by a member of the hospital transfusion committee within a few days of the transfusion having taken place. The results of these reviews were reported at the regular transfusion committee meeting held monthly. If a clinician disagreed with the committee decision, the issue was usually resolved by a "one on one" discussion between the clinician and the transfusion committee chair. If a clinician repeatedly used blood inappropriately, they were reported to their Chief of Service. Ongoing statistics were kept from these reviews; the number of inappropriate transfusion events and the number of units transfused for each different blood component were recorded.

Immediate post-transfusion audit enables rapid feedback to the clinical personnel while the circumstances surrounding a treatment decision are fresh in the memory of the individuals concerned. Although this method does not prevent inappropriate transfusion taking place, continuing education leads in time to a decreased number of inappropriate transfusions.

This form of audit appears to be labour intensive. The San Francisco General Hospital, however, was reported to take only one hour of technologist's time, one hour of the transfusion service resident's time, and only approximately two hours per week for the transfusion service director. Over and above this, the time given by the hospital transfusion committee members for their monthly meeting should be considered, although an estimation of this commitment was not reported. Moreover, many larger, active treatment hospitals do not have transfusion residents or fellows in their institution. They could find this type of evaluation expensive if the work could not be absorbed by the existing staff.

Retrospective audits

This type of audit is performed by abstracting information from the medical records of patients selected after a transfusion either because of their diagnosis [8], the procedure which they had undergone [9], or because they had been transfused with blood products of interest [10]. The review may use isolated transfusion episodes or follow the total transfusion history of the patient. The time limits may include transfusions given over a limited period, a full year or multiple periods. The data that can be collected are varied but usually include: The clinical situation at the time of the decision to transfuse; the relevant laboratory data available to the physician at that time; the request for product that was made; the actual product transfused; the quantity given; and the clinical and laboratory outcomes of the therapy. The thrust of retrospective audits is to determine which transfusions were of doubtful, or of no benefit, to the recipient as judged by a set of pre-determine criteria. By appropriately focusing the review it is possible to determine why certain products were used, how they were used, the transfusion trigger, and to compare the transfusion therapy of different physicians for the same condition.

A retrospective audit can be particularly useful for comparing trends and for determining changing patterns over time. After performing a retrospective review of transfusions given during 1985, we selected three of the sixteen hospitals that were of similar size (300 to 350 beds), that were non-teaching general community hospitals, and had similar quantitative blood product use. We then repeated the review for both red cell and plasma transfusions given during calendar years 1988, and in 1991. The same audit criteria were used for all three evaluations. These had been developed from contemporary literature, especially the consensus conference statements from the National Institute of Health [6]. The criteria were formulated into an algorithm that was used as the tool to abstract information from the hospital medical records. We randomly selected and audited 10% of the red cell transfusion episodes and at least 50% of the plasma transfusion episodes in each of the years audited. For each episode we tried to determine the reason for the transfusion and then designated it as being of clear benefit to the patient, of doubtful benefit, or of no known benefit by comparing it to the previously established criteria. Table 2 summarizes the results for the red cell transfusions over the three audit years. Those considered to have been of benefit increased from 76% to 81% between 1985 and 1991 but with virtually

Table 2. Percentage of red cell transfusions meeting established criteria, versus those of doubtful benefit or no benefit, in each audit year.

Transfusion indicated	Red cells 1985		1988		1991	
Yes	76%		77%		81%	
Doubtful	11%	> 24%	14%	> 23%	16%	> 19%
No	13%		9%		3%	

no change between the 1985 and 1988 audits. Of the remaining transfusion episodes the number of "not-indicated" transfusions decreased quite markedly while those of "doubtful benefit" increased. This probably reflects the concern of the clinicians (or their patients) about the risk of transmissible diseases through the use of blood products.

Three main reasons covered more than half of the "doubtful" and "not-indicated" red cell transfusions in 1985. These were pre-operative transfusions to an asymptomatic elective surgery patient whose hemoglobin was more than 100 g/L; intra-operative transfusion when less than 20% of the blood volume was lost; and post-operative transfusions to asymptomatic patients with a hemoglobin above 100 g/L. By 1988, intra-operative transfusion was the main use

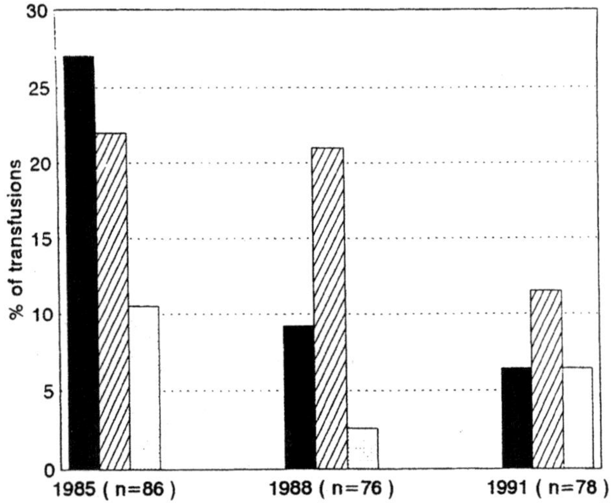

Symbols used:
■ Pre-operative hemoglobin > 100 g/L
▨ Surgical patients with < 20% loss in blood volume
⁞ Post-operative patients with a hemoglobin level > 100 g/L

Figure 1. The three most common reasons for red cell transfusions not meeting established criteria; comparing percentages in the different audit years.

Table 3. Mean pre-transfusion hemoglobin values (g/L) for males and females in each of the three study years.

	1985	1988	1991
Males	107 g/L	102 g/L	99 g/L
Females	97 g/L	96 g/L	89 g/L
n*	350	351	393

* = number of transfusion episodes audited.

and remained so in 1991 although at a much lower percentage (see Figure 1). Of interest, the percentage of pre-operative transfusions actually given to individuals with a hemoglobin above 100 g/L in 1991 (6.4%) matched more closely the percentage of respondents who stated that this would be their practice in the 1985 questionnaire (5%).

These studies also demonstrated a small but steady decline in the mean pre-transfusion hemoglobin of the patients who received red cells, with the trigger in 1991 for both men and women being below the 100 g/L value; a figure that previously had been "carved in stone" (see Table 3). No specific intervention to alter practices had taken place but certainly stricter transfusion criteria were being advocated in the journals and at scientific meetings [11]. In addition, publicity was increasing about the possibility of litigation, especially in the 1989/90 period.

Although there was an increase in appropriate plasma transfusions during the period of study from 37% to 49% it was disappointing to see that these represented less than half of the plasma transfusions administered, even in 1991 (see Table 4). The majority of plasma transfusions were given to bleeding patients and, as can be seen in Figure 2, the proportion of these patients with abnormal coagulation tests increased over time, quite markedly during the three audits.

Of note, plasma given to a patient who had received a massive transfusion was an acceptable criterion. However, on average, these patients did not demonstrate coagulation abnormalities in the prothrombin (PT) and partial thromboplastin (PTT) tests. A smaller percentage of all the plasma transfusions were given to offset a massive transfusion in 1991 (11% as compared with 21% and 28% in 1985 and 1988 respectively), but the most dramatic difference was the increase in the proportion of individuals who had a coagulation test performed

Table 4. Percentage of plasma transfusions meeting established criteria, versus those of doubtful benefit or no benefit, in each audit year.

Transfusion indicated	**Plasma**		
	1985	**1988**	**1991**
Yes	37%	35%	49%
Doubtful	10%	29%	35%
	> 63%	> 65%	> 51%
No	53%	36%	16%

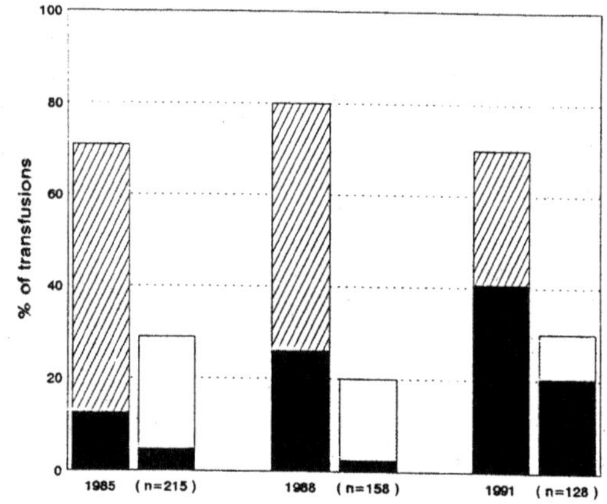

Symbols used:

⁞⁞ Plasma transfusions to patients who were not actively bleeding at the time of transfusion

▨ Plasma transfusions to actively bleeding patients

■ Proportion of patients with abnormal coagulation tests

Figure 2. Percentage of actively bleeding and non-actively bleeding recipients of plasma showing the proportion with abnormal coagulation test results in each of the audit years.

Table 5. Massive transfusion recipients having pre-plasma transfusion coagulation tests performed: Prothrombin time (PT) and partial thromboplastin time (PTT) in the three audit years.

	Normal range	**1985**	**1988**	**1991**
Number of plasma recipients		45	45	14
% of recipients with pre-transfusion tests		29%	60%	88%
Mean PT (secs)	11-14	11.7	11.8	12.3
Mean PTT (secs)	25-42	31.0	28.1	33.5

Table 6. Percentage of patients receiving red cell and/or plasma transfusions in the three study hospitals, in each year audited.

	1985	**1988**	**1991**
Total number of surgical patients	25,266	24,461	24,972
Red cell recipients	9.6%	8.01%	6.8%
Plasma recipients	1.5%	0.8%	0.53%
Total number of non-surgical patients	15,452	18,189	22,874
Red cell recipients	10.4%	7.5%	6.6%
Plasma recipients	0.9%	0.3%	0.3%

pre-transfusion (see Table 5). On the other hand, the results of these tests did not seem to affect the decision to transfuse FFP, as the mean coagulation test results were all within the normal range. Of the 106 coagulation tests performed, 7 were just outside the normal range and only 2 were markedly abnormal (PT 18.1 secs and PTT 83 secs in the same patient in the 1991 audit).

Overall, we noted a decline in the proportion of patients receiving a transfusion. The figures were calculated from the hospital data of the number of acute care discharges and the number of surgical procedures performed per year (see Table 6).

Retrospective review methods are often affected by poor charting; a considerable number of the transfusions designated of doubtful benefit in our studies were so classified because of insufficient information to make a definitive judgement. Correct methods for recording information are considered very important in GMP, the maxim being "if it ain't recorded, it ain't done". This is an area of clinical practice that could benefit greatly by close adherence to the principles of GMP.

Our studies, and practically all those referenced in this chapter, concentrated on the transfused patient. Consideration should be given to the non-transfused patient. To have a true picture of the quality of patient care, omissions should also be noted. We would thus recommend that when a retrospective audit by diagnosis (or procedure) is being performed, the charts of non-transfused patients should be equally reviewed. Non-transfused patients should be evaluated to see whether there was any difference in their speed of recovery or their length of hospital stay compared with the transfused cohort. Were such non-transfused individuals truly at less risk than their transfused fellows? These are unanswered questions at this time.

Any measurement or audit of clinical practice becomes an exercise of limited interest unless some form of follow-up is performed. Inherent to the concurrent review methods is feedback to the physicians. However, the result of this feedback in reducing the inappropriate transfusions met with varying success. Retrospective audits can have little or no impact without the information being given to the appropriate physicians either directly or as general education unless an intervention is devised [12]. One such deliberate intervention was described recently by Soumerai et al. [13]. Using the education approach widely used by pharmaceutical representatives, the intervention devised involved a transfusion specialist giving a 30 minute face-to-face educational outreach visit to each individual physician in the study group. The practices of these physicians six months before and six months after the intervention were measured by a medical chart review as was that of a control group of physicians not receiving the educational visit. There was a statistically significant decline in the number of inappropriate red cell transfusions ordered by the study group of surgeons compared with the surgeons in the control group.

Transfusion Committee

In most jurisdictions in Canada and the USA, hospitals are required to have a Transfusion Committee. The activity of this group varies enormously from that of being very involved with monitoring therapy to that of reviewing single unit transfusions, blood shortages and little else. The committee should be made up of individuals who are respected peers with specialized knowledge related to transfusion medicine. They would thus seem to be the ideal body to establish acceptable criteria, monitor the performance by reviewing audit results and be responsible for direct feedback to physicians. Such a committee would also be a suitable group to recommend or provide ongoing educational programs especially in hospitals without residents and interns. The results of our plasma transfusion audit emphasize that although passive improvement can occur, there is a need for active intervention to change transfusion practices effectively.

In conclusion, we believe that the safety and efficacy of blood component use can be enhanced considerably by the processes outlined in this article. Studies undertaken to compare different forms of therapies for similar procedures, including the non-transfused patient, should allow for a faster resolution of the relative merits of the different transfusion practices. This would enable a definitive re-classification of the indications currently of unproven benefit. Ultimately, the quality of patient care will be enhanced.

Acknowledgements

We thank Dr. J. Lomas of the Department of Clinical Epidemiology and Biostatistics of McMaster University for his assistance with the design of the methodology for this study. We also gratefully acknowledge the Blood Bank and Medical Records Department personnel of all hospitals involved in this study, for their patience and cooperation.

References

1. Lomas J, Anderson GM, Domnick-Pierre K, Vayda E, Enkin M, Hannah WJ. Do practice guidelines guide practice? The effect of a consensus statement on the practice of physicians. N Engl J Med 1989;321:1306-11.
2. Simpson MB. Prospective-concurrent audits and medical consultation for platelet transfusions. Transfusion 1987;27:192-5.
3. Alexander MR, Ambre JJ, Liskow BI, Trost DC. Therapeutic use of albumin. JAMA 1979;241:2527-9.
4. Alexander MR, Alexander B, Mustion AL, Spector R, Wright CB. Therapeutic use of albumin: 2. JAMA 1982;247:831-3.
5. Shanberge JN, Quattrociocchi-Longe T. Analysis of fresh frozen plasma administration with suggestions for ways to reduce usage. Transf Med Rev 1992;2:189-94.
6. National Institutes of Health Consensus Development Conference Statement, 1984. Fresh frozen plasma indications and risks. National Heart, Lung and Blood Institute. Bethesda, Maryland. JAMA 1984;253:551-3.

7. Toy PTCY. Monitoring transfusion practice. In: Kolins J, McCarthy LJ (eds). Contemporary transfusion practice. American Association of Blood Banks, Arlington, VA 1997:85-90.
8. Friedman BA. Patterns of blood utilization by physicians: Transfusion of nonoperated anemic patients. Transfusion 1978;18:193-8.
9. Goodnough LT, Johnston MFM, Toy PTCY and the Transfusion Medicine Academic Award Group. The variability of transfusion practice in coronary artery bypass surgery. JAMA 1991;265:86-90.
10. Ayoub MM, Clark JA. Reduction of fresh frozen plasma use with a simple education program. Am Surg 1989;55:563-5.
11. National Institute of Health Consensus Development Conference, 1988. Perioperative red cell transfusion. National Heart, Lung and Blood Institute, Bethesda, Maryland. Transf Med Rev 1989;1:63-8.
12. Barnette RE, Fish DJ, Eisenstaedt RS. Modification of fresh-frozen plasma transfusion practices through educational intervention. Transfusion 1990;30:253-7.
13. Soumerai SB, Salem-Schatz S, Avorn J, Casteris CS, Ross-Degnan D, Popovsky MA. A controlled trial of educational outreach to improve blood transfusion practice. JAMA 1993;270:961-6.

DISCUSSION

H.J. Heiniger and C.Th. Smit Sibinga

A. Heaton (San Francisco, CA, USA): Dr. Wells, in terms of auditing I noticed that you focused only upon the issue of the pharmaceutical manufacturer auditing their clinical investigator. Presumably the pharmaceutical manufacturers submit their clinical data to a licensing agency similar to the United States Food and Drug Administration. Does the UK licensing agency routinely or randomly audit these clinical investigators independent of the pharmaceutical manufacturer?

F. Wells (London, UK): The short answer is: Certainly in the United States this happens, where the FDA conducts site audits. In Europe the situation is currently being established. In France and in Germany there is in place an inspectorate of the licensing authority. In the United Kingdom it is being discussed how that inspectorate should actually be set up. In my view it is very important that there is an independent audit function of the licensing authority as indeed is provided by the FDA.

A. Heaton: I noticed that your guidelines do not have a requirement, specifying that if there are new valuable findings discovered as a result of the research, that these should be communicated to the research participants. In many cases the motivation for the research participant will be the acquisition of knowledge about a new drug or acquisition of treatment. In the United States it is standard now to provide any recent information to participants in trials as part of the "Right to Know" for participating in the trial. Is that the same in the UK?

F. Wells: It is not as firmly defined as that, but it is something that I personally strongly support, and which is going to be more and more required as an expectation by research ethics committees. I think the patient has every right to know what is happening to him and has a right of interest to know what happened to the product in which he was involved. I have to respect commercial confidentiality and it may be sometime before it is appropriate that I should have that information. Yes, it is something that is right and proper and that I would support.

C.Th. Smit Sibinga (Groningen, NL): Dr. Klazinga, a question related to what Dr. Hannema was providing us as information in relation to the new regulations in the Netherlands, where blood transfusion in the hospital has to be documented and will in a short period of time become effective. That might dramatically further effect the organization in the set up and the filling in of responsibilities of the blood transfusion practice in the clinic. Is CBO aware of that and if so has CBO in mind an evaluation on a consensus basis to monitor the effects of the implementation of this new regulation?

N.S. Klazinga (Utrecht, NL): Well, we are aware of that. There are of course different types of regulations. One of the major ones we are now looking at is the new regulation on Quality Assurance in health care institutions. That type of regulation in the Netherlands is very general, because the general policy of the government is that they want to get rid of very detailed regulations, but they want to stimulate the development of quality systems in hospitals. So, that is the central element in the new law on quality systems in hospitals. Apart from that, there exists on the quality of blood products specific regulation. What I also tried to demonstrate in my presentation is, that you should try to establish a good link between the Good Manufacturing Practice of the blood and the quality systems that are now being built and being enforced in the hospitals. As CBO is a support organization, we have no authority in saying what should be done. What we try to do is to develop those mechanisms. We work very intensely on the implementation of the national guidelines through the scientific associations and the audit committees. However, we are thinking about doing a second evaluation on the red blood cell transfusion, because it was revised in 1989. That means in our own procedures that we have to revise the whole text again in 1994. I think it would be a good idea to have a new evaluation to see if practices have changed dramatically since the evaluation we performed in 1989.

B.T. Teague (Houston, TX, USA): Dr. Klazinga, first I compliment you on your efforts to implement your Quality Assurance program. My question is: From your perspective how can a regional blood center assist you in getting those programs implemented in the individual hospital.

N.S. Klazinga: Well, there are different ways. One is of course the anticipation in the guideline setting process and that was surely no problem in the past. The blood banks, the regional centers are aware of these problems and they come up with all kind of ideas to help to improve. The second is of course through the heads of the laboratories, because they are more the key persons for introducing changes in the hospital. That has a lot to do with their credibility in the hospital and their ability to discuss with the physicians these kind of things. So, in a way the CBO and regional blood bank centers are doing the same in the direction of hospitals: Both trying to support and stimulate better practice. It is good to keep communicating so that we both stimulate and develop in the same direction.

H.J. Heiniger (Bern, CH): Dr. de Wolf, you mentioned very appropriately the situation of standards, guidelines and options in clinical practice. What is, at present, the relative distribution. How many areas are covered by standards, how many areas are covered by guidelines and what is still completely open. So, what is the distribution of standards versus guidelines versus options?

J.Th.M. de Wolf (Groningen, NL): I think that most practice policies fall in the category of guidelines. In guidelines from NIH or from The Netherlands, there is missing an overview of the evidence which led to the proposed intervention and most of all is missing alternatives. The point is that in a clinical guideline it should start with the patient. We try to improve the health care of the patient. It is to the patient to decide what is an acceptable risk for him or not. Many guidelines, practice policies, miss those points.

I. Helsper (Utrecht, NL): The inappropriate use you mentioned, is that use when products should not be used, mainly?

J.Th.M. de Wolf: That is true.

I. Helsper: Then it would mean that twice as much blood products are used than there should be according to the guidelines.

J.Th.M. de Wolf: That is true. That concerns plasma but also albumin. Also for the guidelines for albumin it misses the alternatives, the plasma expanders, which you can use instead of albumin. I think that for many hospitals, also in the Netherlands, 80 to 90 per cent of the plasma and albumin products are used unnecessarily where there are good alternatives.

H. Bremer (Eindhoven, NL): During this symposium, I listened carefully to what is in your minds; where are you on the scale from inspection to fully implemented people oriented TQM? In Figure 1 I give my best estimation. On the horizontal axis is the time scale, indicating that, as an average, it will take some ten years to transfer an organization from a Taylor/inspection into a TQM culture. In such a time span, many things have to be changed, e.g.:

- The profile of the managers from the (present) Taylor-managers into leaders.
- Audits, now mainly carried out by third parties, to be carried out by the president and/or colleagues, the so-called peer audits.
- There are a number of stages to go through: Inspection, QC, QA, quality management, quality improvement, organization structuring and last but not least, one will arrive at the TQM level.
- The defects/failure culture will move from 0/0 via 0/00 to close to zero-defects level, defects are expressed in Parts Per Million (PPM).
- Costs will increase slightly in the very beginning as one has to invest in education and training and help from other parties, but will definitely decrease after a certain period of time.

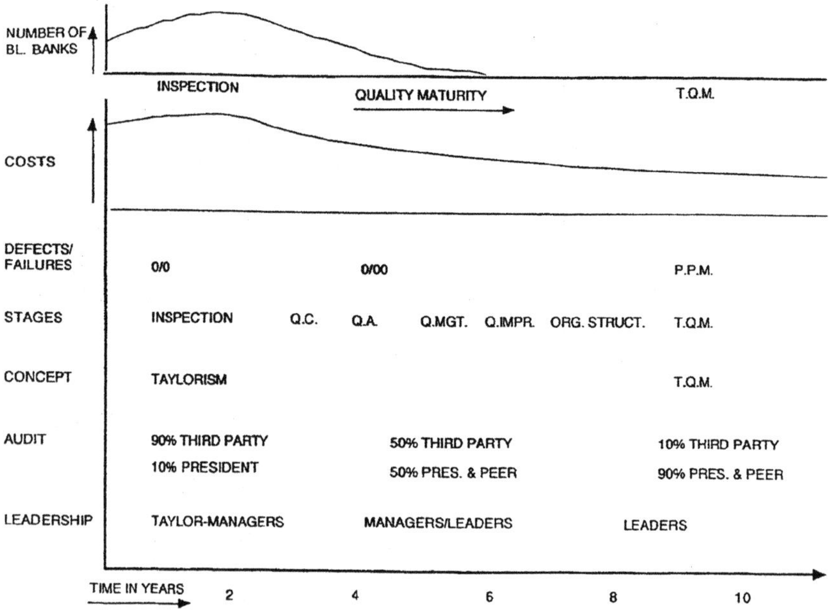

Figure 1.

Based on my experience in other fields than blood banks, combined with the information from many of you during the coffeebreaks/lunches etc. And, of course, from the many excellent presentations I heard, I can convey to you two good messages:

- Quite a number of you here present have started up quality activities in the right way!
- While you all have much room for further improvement, there is appreciation of a real challenge!

In Figure 1, I have also indicated the position of the blood banks as my best estimation.

F. Wells: Chairman, I very much would like to comment on the nice things I have heard with very great interest. I might have given the impression that these things were effectively rules which just existed. All the things you have talked about emphasize how enormously important it is to communicate and discuss with others and I am sure Dr. de Wolf will confirm this. If you have actually got an agreement amongst the people who are doing it themselves as to what these new guidelines should be, you can achieve them. If we had not involved them early enough in deciding what these rules should be, how could we expect them to be involved in fulfilling them?

J.Th.M. de Wolf: That is right. I think that doctors change their behaviour, when they see what the profit will be for patients. When there are guidelines in general and you form indications for blood products, you can hear from many doctors: Well my experience, you may be right but I had a patient and so on.

T.E. Warkentin (Hamilton, C): Dr. Smit Sibinga, what you showed in a previous slide is the assumption that adherence to total quality management in GMP results in a decrease in transfusion-related morbidity and mortality. I would like to challenge that assumption. When I think of the complications that we see in transfusion medicine, ranging from mild ones (such as febrile transfusion reactions or urticaria) to more morbid ones (such as delayed hemolytic transfusion reactions that occur despite initial negative serum screening) or to life-threatening complications (such as hepatitis C or the AIDS problem – which can continue to occur because of the "window period" prior to the detection of HIV IgG), it seems to me that a large majority of transfusion-related morbidity and mortality will continue to happen, and will require ongoing scientific measures to try to understand and try to improve upon them. However, these kind of measures (GMP) will not have any significant impact, and I want to hear your comments on that point.

C.Th. Smit Sibinga: It is always good to be challenged. However, I do not think I can agree on your challenge. The principle of TQM as we discussed it over these days is in the community from which our source material, the human blood as a tissue comes: Start improving your efforts first in the information and the education of the public and lead that through the whole processing and quality controlling procedures in the blood bank right into the clinic where an immense amount of education needs to be done. I think we can see (we already have seen in this country) a definite drop in the mortality but also in the morbidity. Of course, transfusion risks will remain. There is no such a thing like zero risk as we tried to discuss, because if you want a zero risk you should avoid the exposure and that is kind of a difficulty, because every once in a while there might be a need for exposure. So, if you want to avoid that, you should try to come to non-existence. That is another problem, how do we get to non-existence? The only way to get to that is not being borne and unfortunately that is not in our hands. So, there will always be a risk and you are right in that respect, but the magnitude both quantitatively as well as qualitatively will definitely be influenced if we do our jobs correct and in a well defined manner: Total Quality Management.

J. Verburg (Hoogeveen, NL): What I am missing in the CBO consensus is the place of the patient. I think it is rather important. Compared to other subjects like giving or prescribing medicines and the decisions to operate the information to the patients is very poor in the area of blood transfusion. We could hear that from Dr. McClelland and also from Dr. Ali. I have two questions. What do you think about an obligation of information to the patient about a possible transfusion and the risks of it, and what do you think about the possibility of reaching in certain cases a better and more specific ordering and transfusion prescription by also discussing the transfusion indication with the patient and providing a certain information about the risks of transfusion?

F. Wells: Obviously I am not qualified to talk about blood transfusion at all, but I am qualified to talk about information to patients. I think it is now enormously important that patients have as much information as they want and as much information as is available (if they want it) about the pros and cons of taking medicines. I would extend that to the pros and cons of receiving blood. There are some regulations which exist now in the pharmaceutical world, which require information to be made available for patients about drugs. We have discussed this with, particularly, oncologists and psychiatrists, because there was concern that it might not be appropriate for patients with cancer and patients with severe mental illness to have information about their medicines. But there is overwhelming support from the specialists concerned and above all from patients organizations that this information should be available. It should be the norm that they have this information. I believe that it should be the same with blood.

J.Th.M. de Wolf: Yes, I think it is necessary. I think every guideline should include estimations about the outcomes which you have to discuss with the patient. Every guideline should also contain or discuss alternatives: What are the harms and benefits and these should also be discussed with the patient.

A. Heaton: I think that this is an important area since for some years I have been much involved in running a large research licensing laboratory in the United States that performs the studies required to license new products, or methods, or processing of blood products. One of the best aspects of the US FDA system is, that there is a very carefully controlled program, which requires clinical research to validate not only the drug or the product, but also the conditions of manufacturing and the conditions of use. For example, we would license red cells that must be manufactured within so many hours of phlebotomy in a specified fashion. Yet I notice that in Europe it is common practice to allow manufacturers to secure registration of blood products without doing radio-isotope studies to verify whether the red cells are really effective. This can lead to difficulties since these studies are the only definitive measure of red cell quality. For example, we have just finished a study showing that if you separate red cells after a 24 hour period of 22°C hold, you get slightly reduced post transfusion recoveries. This method appears to be common practice in the European literature yet there appears to be no licensing data to support such a manufacturing change. A practical question I would, therefore, raise for you is to whether you believe it is appropriate to not only regulate the licensing of drug, but also to regulate the detailed manufacturing process since there appears to be more latitude in the European regulations in this area.

F. Wells: Certainly in the context of manufacturing of medicines there are very clear GMP guidelines, which preceded GLP (good laboratory) guidelines and GCP guidelines. I do not know about the manufacture of blood related products, but certainly where pharmaceutical products are concerned it is essential that there are clear guidelines, which have the effect of rules in this particular context, on the manufacture of the finished product.

A. Heaton: The other question or observation that I would like to make to Dr. de Wolf relates to the effectiveness of the application of consensus standards to clinical practice in the United States. In the United States as you commented it took some time before the consensus guidelines of the NIH became effective in the clinical world. I think three things really greatly influenced that. The first was the guidelines were merely guidelines and they achieved little change on their own. What achieved the change was the high price of failure to follow the guidelines. If you get sued for failing to follow the guidelines, it is very expensive. Compared to Europe it is much more expensive in the USA not to follow guidelines and that certainly was one big determinant to secure rapid change.

The second issue was that we often assign medical staff to visit hospital transfusion committees and to provide guidance to them. For example, I routinely attended Dr. Toy's Transfusion Committee, at the University of California, San Francisco Medical School, and therefore, the blood center participates with the hospital in the decision making process. This helps influence clinical behaviour and results in a responsive blood center.

The third issue is cost. We have tremendous pressure on cost at present and probably the biggest reason for change or modification is a desire on the part of the administration to greatly cut the costs of healthcare. So, I think it is unfair to say that the NIH guidelines were ineffective. I think they were very effective, but you need the composite of risk, cost, advice and guidance in order to achieve the outcome, that you would like to see.

J.Th.M. de Wolf: I am not very happy that the guidelines became effective in the way you describe it, because it is in my view not very important to use as less as possible of a certain product. There are a few shortcomings on those consensus conferences. If you talk about albumin or plasma, you should not talk only about plasma and albumin; you should talk and tell the doctor what he should use as an alternative. You should also look at outcome: The patient who does not get the product, is he better off or worse? What happens with those patients? For me it is not only cost containment, I think it is quality of the patients' treatment.

K. Sazama (Sacramento, USA): I would like to make one comment and then ask a question. I completely agree with Dr. Wells regarding the patient's right to have information. This right has been translated in the state of California into mandatory information sheet and documented discussion.

My question is really for Drs. de Wolf and Ali. In all published audits of transfusion practice, there seems to be a rather simplistic view. By that comment

I mean that red cell use is audited as if every red cell transfused is exactly identical. Back to Dr. Heaton's comment, in fact, the complexity of the transfusion choices available in 1993 suggest that perhaps the audits have not begun to accomplish all of good clinical practice. Just a simple illustration in the US, certainly in our region, the issue of what to do about removing white blood cells from red cell units is not settled. Also, every red cell unit differs by its anticoagulant, additive or preservative solution. Therefore, not every red cell component is equivalent. I just wonder if you like to comment about how extensive the audit should be. Should we just be focusing on red cells compared with platelets or should we be looking at the nature and type of the red cell, how it is prepared and what its ultimate goal is.

A.M. Ali (Hamilton, C): I think at the moment we are still at the very early stages and consequently we do take the simplistic view. Certainly looking at chart reviews we can only say this is what was given and have some idea about why. In Canada we have only one set of individuals, manufacturers if you like, producing the product. Consequently, it is a fairly similar type of product and the clinician does not have the choice between whether they have red cells that had additive or CPDA-1 or some other preservative. White cell removal certainly may not be recorded and, of course, all of this is going to be very important within the quality of care. But going back to the simplistic stage, still quite a lot of products are given where it is probably not necessary to give them. The question of whether there are patients who should have had products who have not, is not known, and that is something that has to be answered. Certainly from some of the work where physicians have a large practice with Jehovah's Witnesses, they have found that a lot of treatments and procedures can be done without blood and without apparent increase in hospital stay, increase or delay in wound healing or any of the other "reasons" for which we sometimes give transfusions. I think we have got a long way to go.

C.Th. Smit Sibinga: Dr. Sazama, there is a difference between an audit as described by Dr. Ali and what you really are looking for, which is more something for a survey or even a clinical trial to find out how the efficacy of individual products is and how the standardization therefore of product should be before one comes to a general audit. You need two separate issues.

K. Sazama: I can agree in part with your comment, but I think it is also a very common practice, for example in the use of platelets, for variations to be extreme. One can use platelets obtained by whole blood donation or apheresis that are medically-designated, HLA-matched, random or crossmatch-comparable. All of these platelet components are audited as if they are interchangeable. When one considers some of the conditions that Dr. Heaton illustrated in terms of the cost/benefit and resource availability, these are not equivalent therapies. In terms of auditing, by what criteria should evaluations be made? One cannot afford to simply consider every single component as exactly identical.

J.A. van der Does ('s-Gravenhage, NL): In all the presentations it came out that it is very important that the clinicians in the hospital decide what their standards are, what they want to do. Whether it is derived within that hospital or from national consensus meetings. The problem I encounter and when I talk with colleagues they encounter it as well, is that the laboratory people in the hospitals are quite willing to set standards, to make decisions on formal protocols, but that doctors are much less inclined to do so. Now, even if you start with a few guidelines in the hospital, which you can audit then you have a starting point. However, in some hospitals the clinicians say: No, we do not want to make standard requirements or guidelines. I would like Dr. Ali and Dr. de Wolf to comment on how to approach hospitals to start somewhere in that area.

J.Th.M. de Wolf: I do not know. My remark was that we have to learn very much about why doctors treat their patients the way they do. There is a lot of medicine that is called science, but there is little science on patient care. Therefore we need to know more about the factors that lead to a change in the clinical behaviour. Until that time it is trial and error, I think.

A.M. Ali: I have not had the need to do this. I mean that I am in the fortunate position that I am not within the hospital and working with a group of clinicians. From the literature it looks as if it is a lot of hard work by repeatedly going to the clinicians who are using the products that you may consider inappropriate and explaining to them why, and have them tell you why they used it. It will take time, but if the guidelines are there at least that is something to begin with: Then you have to have constant one on one type meetings with those individuals who do not like the criteria.

D.B.L. McClelland (Edinburgh, UK): Chairman, if I can make two brief comments, I would be grateful. Number one: Coming back to Dr. Sazama's point of unnecessary transfusions, we have heard briefly of the SANGUIS study of patients in Europe having elective surgery. One of the very clear results of that study, involving 5000 adult elective surgical patients who did receive red cell transfusion, is that 50 per cent of those patients received one or more red cell unit, that brought their hemoglobin above a level of 11 grams. Many patients received more than one unit of red cells, apparently in excess of obvious need. In fact, of the total red cell units administer to those 5000 patients, 53 per cent fell into the category of probably not necessary, even by generous criteria.

The second comment goes back to Dr. Heaton's and Dr. Sazama's point. The product that we are auditing is extremely non-standard in the most elementary property, which is that it contains between a 140 and 250 ml of red cells. So, a dose can vary by 60-70 per cent; that is never taken into account.

R. Schuurmans (de Bilt, NL): Mr. Bremer, do you see a possibility to shift that maximum more to the right, more to the TQM? As I understood, it was mainly the "fit for use", which was important in any step of the process or of the product as a whole. The use for a product is determined by guidelines, which can be viewed upon very differently: In a legal sense, as Dr. Heaton just brought up or in a quality sense. So, if the use is determined by guidelines, what is the optimal "fit for use"? How can we then shift that maximum to the right?

H. Bremer: Thank you for your question. As in many Taylor-oriented organizations, TQM is now a far away goal, and as long as the ideas of "fit for use" are not practised within an organization (internal supplier-customer relations) and other concepts related to TQM are still missing, one must rely on standards and a rigid third party audit system. If an organization operates, however, according to the people oriented TQM concept, the internal suppliers will deliver "fit for use" products, in the widest sense, to their internal customers both in a legal as well as in a quality sense. The need for rigid prescriptions and tough auditing decreases strongly. However, in the case of blood products, at all times one must be prepared to be able to demonstrate that system standards used will guarantee the purity of the blood and blood products. TQM – the concept of "fit for use" throughout the organization – can only enhance this requirement at the lowest costs!

Index

DEVELOPMENTS IN HEMATOLOGY AND IMMUNOLOGY

1. H.R. Lijnen, D. Collen and M. Verstraete (eds.): *Synthetic Substrates in Clinical Blood Coagulation Assays*. 1980 ISBN 90-247-2409-0
2. C.Th. Smit Sibinga, P.C. Das and J.O. Forfar (eds.): *Paediatrics and Blood Transfusion*. Proceedings of the 5th Annual Symposium on Blood Transfusion, organized by the Red Cross Bloodbank Groningen-Drenthe, The Netherlands (1980). 1982 ISBN 90-247-2619-0
3. N. Fabris (ed.): *Immunology and Ageing*. 1982 ISBN 90-247-2640-9
4. G. Hornstra: *Dietary Fats, Prostanoids and Arterial Thrombosis*. With an Introductory Chapter by A. Bleakley Chandler. 1982 ISBN 90-247-2667-0
5. C.Th. Smit Sibinga, P.C. Das and J.J. van Loghem (eds.): *Blood Transfusion and Problems of Bleeding*. Proceedings of the 6th Annual Symposium on Blood Transfusion, organized by the Red Cross Bloodbank Groningen-Drenthe (1981). 1982 ISBN 90-247-3058-9
6. J. Dormandy (ed.): *Red Cell Deformability and Filterability*. 1983 ISBN 0-89838-578-4
7. C.Th. Smit Sibinga, P.C. Das and H.F. Taswell (eds.): *Quality Assurance in Blood Banking and Its Clinical Impact*. Proceedings of the 7th Annual Symposium on Blood Transfusion, organized by the Red Cross Bloodbank Groningen-Drenthe (1982). 1984 ISBN 0-89838-618-7
8. A.M.H.P. van den Besselaar, H.R. Gralnick and S.M. Lewis (eds.): *Thromboplastin Calibration and Oral Anticoagulant Control*. 1984 ISBN 0-89838-637-3
9. P. Fondu and O. Thijs (eds.): *Haemostatic Failure in Liver Disease*. 1984 ISBN 0-89838-640-3
10. C.Th. Smit Sibinga, P.C. Das and G. Opelz (eds.): *Transplantation and Blood Transfusion*. Proceedings of the 8th Annual Symposium on Blood Transfusion, organized by the Red Cross Bloodbank Groningen-Drenthe (1983). 1984 ISBN 0-89838-686-1
11. H. Schmid-Schönbein, L.J. Wurzinger and R.E. Zimmerman (eds.): *Enzyme Activation in Blood-perfused Artificial Organs*. 1985 ISBN 0-89838-704-3
12. J. Dormandy (ed.): *Blood Filtration and Blood Cell Deformability*. 1985 ISBN 0-89838-714-0
13. C.Th. Smit Sibinga, P.C. Das and E. Seidl (eds.): *Plasma Fractionation and Blood Transfusion*. Proceedings of the 9th Annual Symposium on Blood Transfusion, organized by the Red Cross Bloodbank Groningen-Drenthe (1984). 1985 ISBN 0-89838-761-2
14. S. Dawids and A. Bantjes (eds.): *Blood Compatible Materials and their Testing*. 1986 ISBN 0-89838-813-9
15. C.Th. Smit Sibinga, P.C. Das and T.J. Greenwalt (eds.): *Future Developments in Blood Banking*. Proceedings of the 10th Annual Symposium on Blood Transfusion, organized by the Red Cross Bloodbank Groningen-Drenthe (1985). 1986 ISBN 0-89838-824-4
16. A. Berlin, J. Dean, M.H. Draper, E.M.B. Smith and F. Spreafico (eds.): *Immunotoxicology*. Proceedings of the International Seminar on the Immunological System as a Target for Toxic Damage – Present Status, Open Problems and Future Perspectives, in collaboration with the UNEP-ILO-WHO IPCS and the Commission of the European Communities. 1987 ISBN 0-89838-843-0

DEVELOPMENTS IN HEMATOLOGY AND IMMUNOLOGY

17. T. Ottenhoff and R. de Vries: *Recognition of M. leprae Antigens.* 1987
ISBN 0-89838-887-2
18. J.-L. Touraine, R.P. Gale and V. Kochupillai (eds.): *Fetal Liver Transplantation.* 1987
ISBN 0-89838-975-5
19. C.Th. Smit Sibinga P.C. Das and C.P. Engelfriet (eds.): *White Cells and Platelets in Blood Transfusion.* Proceedings of the 11th Annual Symposium on Blood Transfusion, organized by the Red Cross Bloodbank Groningen-Drenthe (1986). 1987
ISBN 0-89838-976-3
20. C.F.M. Hendriksen: *Laboratory Animals in Vaccine Production and Control.* 1988
ISBN 0-89838-398-6
21. C.Th. Smit Sibinga, P.C. Das and L.R. Overby (eds.): *Biotechnology in Blood Transfusion.* Proceedings of the 12th Annual Symposium on Blood Transfusion, organized by the Red Cross Bloodbank Groningen-Drenthe (1987). 1988
ISBN 0-89838-404-4
22. C.Th. Smit Sibinga, P.C. Das and C.F. Högman (eds.): *Automation in Blood Transfusion.* Proceedings of the 13th Annual Symposium on Blood Transfusion, organized by the Red Cross Bloodbank Groningen-Drenthe (1988). 1989
ISBN 0-7923-0488-8
23. S. Dawids (ed.): *Polymers: Their Properties and Blood Compatibility.* 1989
ISBN 0-7923-0491-8
24. C.Th. Smit Sibinga, P.C. Das and H.T. Meryman (eds.): *Cryopreservation and Low Temperature Biology in Blood Transfusion.* Proceedings of the 14th Annual Symposium on Blood Transfusion, organized by the Red Cross Bloodbank Groningen-Drenthe (1989). 1990 ISBN 0-7923-0908-1
25. C.Th. Smit Sibinga and L. Kater (eds.): *Advances in Haemapheresis.* Proceedings of the 3rd International Congress of the World Apheresis Association (Amsterdam, The Netherlands, 1990). 1991 ISBN 0-7923-1312-7
26. C.Th. Smit Sibinga, P.C. Das and P.M. Mannucci (eds.): *Coagulation and Blood Transfusion.* Proceedings of the 15th Annual Symposium on Blood Transfusion, organized by the Red Cross Bloodbank Groningen-Drenthe (1990). 1991
ISBN 0-7923-1331-3
27. C.Th. Smit Sibinga, P.C. Das and J.D. Cash (eds.): *Transfusion Medicine: Fact and Fiction.* Proceedings of the 16th International Symposium on Blood Transfusion, organized by the Red Cross Bloodbank Groningen-Drenthe (1991). 1992
ISBN 0-7923-1732-7
28. C.Th. Smit Sibinga, P.C. Das and T.H. The (eds.): *Immunology and Blood Transfusion.* Proceedings of the 17th International Symposium on Blood Transfusion, organized by the Red Cross Bloodbank Groningen-Drenthe (1992). 1993
ISBN 0-7923-2380-7
29. C.Th. Smit Sibinga, P.C. Das and H.J. Heiniger (eds.): *Good Manufacturing Practice in Transfusion Medicine.* Proceedings of the 18th International Symposium on Blood Transfusion, organized by the Red Cross Blood Bank Groningen-Drenthe. (1993) 1994 ISBN 0-7923-3009-9

KLUWER ACADEMIC PUBLISHERS – DORDRECHT / BOSTON / LONDON

GPSR Compliance

The European Union's (EU) General Product Safety Regulation (GPSR) is a set of rules that requires consumer products to be safe and our obligations to ensure this.

If you have any concerns about our products, you can contact us on ProductSafety@springernature.com

In case Publisher is established outside the EU, the EU authorized representative is:

Springer Nature Customer Service Center GmbH
Europaplatz 3
69115 Heidelberg, Germany

Batch number: 10755284

Printed by Printforce, the Netherlands